"What could be more important than protecting the health of those who serve our country and defend us all? In doing that important task, what could be more essential than remaining open minded and yet critically minded toward new possibilities? We need people who embrace the new, who train themselves to grasp the unfamiliar, who do not see AI as intrinsically a threat nor intrinsically a godsend that will solve all our problems. Professor Hassan Tetteh is such a scholar. He evaluates AI's potential as a powerful tool and does so with the hard mind of a rock-solid scientific thinker."

—David B. Allison, PhD
Academic dean and distinguished professor

"Dr. Hassan Tetteh's *Smarter Healthcare with AI* brilliantly bridges the gap between cutting-edge technology and heartfelt human care. With keen insights and visionary foresight, this book is essential for anyone seeking to explore how AI can enhance the future of healthcare through compassion and innovation."

—Gil Alterovitz, PhD, FACMI, FAMIA
Harvard Medical Faculty

"Dr. Tetteh gets it! He truly understands the future of healthcare. Smarter healthcare is crucial for maintaining a strong global military presence and revolutionizing medicine beyond the battlefield. Having served with him, I can attest to his exceptional vision, dedication, and mentorship. This book brilliantly explores the history of military medicine, AI-driven suicide prevention, and ethical considerations, addressing critical topics and offering a visionary framework for the future of healthcare. It's an inspiring and transformative read for anyone passionate about challenging the status quo and gaining insight into the unique career of a military physician."

—Roger Boodoo, MD
Defense Health Agency Innovation

"It is said that, in war, the only victor is medicine. Military healthcare has always been at the forefront of medicine and medical innovation, committed to honoring the trust placed in our hands to provide our service members with the best care our nation can offer and from which others will also benefit. AI, the hallmark advancement of our time, can do much to ensure we continue to honor that trust. Dr. Tetteh has masterfully laid out a plan and road map that will ensure AI delivers on its promise and opportunity to transform healthcare, both for our service members and for all patients. A must read for all medical leaders and for anyone committed to ensuring that, today and tomorrow, the patient and the best care we can provide are at the center of all we do."

—C. Forrest Faison III, MD, ScD, FAAP
Vice Admiral (retired), Medical Corps, US Navy | 38th Surgeon General, US Navy

"I am thoroughly impressed by Dr. Hassan Tetteh's *Smarter Healthcare with AI*. Dr. Tetteh's deep understanding of AI's transformative potential in healthcare is unparalleled. His visions for leveraging AI include not only enhancing patient care but also creating a way to democratize access to cutting-edge medical advancements. Using his innovative VP4 framework and drawing from his extensive experience as a heart and lung surgeon and as an AI strategist, Dr. Tetteh provides invaluable insights into creating a more personalized, efficient, and equitable healthcare system. This book is an essential read for anyone seeking to harness the power of AI to drive the future of medicine forward."

—Meghan E. Gilson, MEd, MSE
CEO, Nexus Impact Services | Instructor, University of Arizona Global Campus

"In *Smarter Healthcare with AI*, Dr. Tetteh brilliantly merges his profound experience in AI and healthcare with his unique expertise as a heart surgeon and leader in the military. His lucid and engaging writing makes complex AI concepts accessible as he bridges the gap between technical expertise and practical applications. Dr. Tetteh presents a pioneering vision and offers a road map that will undoubtedly shape the future of healthcare, making his book a 'must read' for all who aspire to harness the power of AI to improve the future of medicine."

—Robert L. Gordon III
Senior AI strategist | Former Deputy Undersecretary of Defense (MCFP)

"Dr. Hassan Tetteh masterfully bridges the gap between military medicine and the transformative power of artificial intelligence in his groundbreaking book, *Smarter Healthcare with AI: Harnessing Military Medicine to Revolutionize Health-care for Everyone, Everywhere.* With a visionary approach, Dr. Tetteh offers a comprehensive road map that not only underscores the profound potential of AI in healthcare but also emphasizes the importance of compassionate care. His insights are deeply rooted in real-world examples, making this work both compelling and inspiring. As a leader who has witnessed the evolution of healthcare firsthand, I find Dr. Tetteh's unique perspective and deep expertise invaluable. This book is an essential read for healthcare professionals, tech enthusiasts, and anyone passionate about the future of healthcare. Dr. Tetteh's pioneering vision will undoubtedly shape the future of medicine, making this a must-read for all."

—Elder Granger, MD
Major General (retired), US Army | President and CEO, 5Ps LLC | Former deputy director, TRICARE Management Activity (TMA)

"Dr. Hassan Tetteh offers a visionary, inspiring, and practical road map for harnessing the immense power of AI to make healthcare both more effective and more humane. With his extensive medical, military, and AI experience, he is the perfect guide. He is also a very fine writer, and he threads the book with the story of his remarkable personal journey. Highly recommended."

—John Hagelin
President, Maharishi International University | International director, Global Union of Scientists for Peace

"Dr. Hassan Tetteh's latest work is a tour de force. With remarkable clarity, candor, and compassion, he cogently describes the enormous potential for combining human ingenuity with artificial intelligence (AI) to heal people everywhere. Grounded in Dr. Tetteh's keen insights as a skilled surgeon and visionary strategist, his powerful VP4 framework embraces a truly human-centered approach for integrating AI into healthcare systems around the world. If you want an inspiring glimpse of humanity's future and a realistic road map for how to design and deploy AI to save lives and alleviate suffering, then read *Smarter Healthcare with AI*."

—Amol M. Joshi, PhD, MS, MBA
Thomas H. Davis Professor in Business
Wake Forest University School of Business and School of Medicine

"In *Smarter Healthcare with AI*, Dr. Hassan Tetteh makes a compelling case that the military must embrace AI to improve the healthcare we provide to the men and women of the Armed Forces. Drawing on his decades of experience as a surgeon and a leader of the Joint Artificial Intelligence Center, Dr. Tetteh provides a road map for using AI to reduce code blues and save lives."

—Tom Kalil
CEO, Renaissance Philanthropy

"Called the 'Unicorn' due to his unique ability to observe, learn, and create innovative healthcare solutions using AI,

Dr. Hassan Tetteh applies his global military knowledge with his medical expertise in this book as an informative tool aimed at making this world a better, healthier place to live for everyone."

—Fred Katz
Senior professional faculty, Johns Hopkins University Carey Business School

"With an exemplary bedside manner that puts everyone at ease, Dr. Hassan Tetteh has saved many lives and transformed patients' quality of post-surgical life—both on the chaotic battlefield and in quiet operating rooms over the course of his accomplished career. In an easy-to-grasp, relatable manner, Dr. Tetteh now describes the framework and future of AI to improve healthcare and enhance the healing hands of future healthcare professionals in *Smarter Healthcare with AI: Harnessing Military Medicine to Revolutionize Healthcare for Everyone, Everywhere*. His book is enjoyable, enlightening, and educational—something we have come to expect from the incomparable Dr. Tetteh. His experience and intensity are easy to admire, but I could also imagine his broad smile and friendly bedside manner while reading his latest book."

—Steven Munatones
CEO and cofounder, KAATSU Global Inc.

"Dr. Hassan Tetteh recognizes the amazing present and future capability of AI in transforming accessibility, diagnosis, treatment, and accelerated learning for healthcare. In his book *Smarter Healthcare with AI: Harnessing Military Medicine to*

Revolutionize Healthcare for Everyone, Everywhere, Dr. Tetteh combines his passion for clinical care, medical informatics, and a distinguished military career to help novice and expert alike better navigate and target efforts where AI can and will impact healthcare providers and patients. He highlights the unique capabilities and challenges in military healthcare to offer blueprints, imperatives, as well as warnings in the midst of an AI technocracy that has just begun to influence and at times dominate so many aspects of our lives. For those who feel overwhelmed with the fact and fiction of AI and are looking for a road map to organize their approach and understanding of the way ahead, this book is required reading."

—Matthew L. Nathan, MD, FACP
Vice Admiral (retired), Medical Corps, US Navy | 37th Surgeon General, US Navy

"As artificial intelligence (AI) becomes increasingly integrated into various industries, from social media to education, concerns about its rapid adoption are inevitable, particularly in the healthcare sector. The promise of AI in healthcare is immense, but so are the potential pitfalls, especially regarding the loss of the personal touch that is crucial in patient care. Enter Dr. Hassan Tetteh's latest book, *Smarter Healthcare with AI,* a timely and insightful exploration of this technological frontier. With his unique blend of experience as a patient, a thoracic surgeon, a military physician, and a leader in medical informatics, Dr. Tetteh offers a balanced perspective on the application of AI in healthcare. His writing is a breath of fresh air, combining the artistry of human care with the precision of artificial intelligence.

In *Smarter Healthcare with AI*, Dr. Tetteh not only highlights AI's transformative potential but also candidly addresses its limitations and the concerns it raises. This masterfully written book is a must read for anyone interested in the future of healthcare. It seamlessly blends the art and science of medicine, providing a comprehensive guide to understanding and navigating the integration of AI in healthcare."

—Roger A. Orsini, MD, MBA, FACS
Surgeon

"Dr. Hassan Tetteh artfully connects the realm of endless possibilities to join artificial intelligence and military medicine. These two powerful fields will revolutionize healthcare delivery. By leveraging precision, efficiency, and predictive capabilities, Dr. Tetteh's vision paves the way for a healthcare system that is more responsive, resilient, and equitable. This book not only represents a call to action; it is a blueprint for transforming global healthcare, placing emphasis on harnessing cutting-edge technologies to save lives, improve outcomes, and deliver unparalleled care and hope to all. This is essential reading for healthcare professionals, policymakers, and innovators!"

—Michelle Padgett, MA, LPC, NCC, CFLE
Former director, Warfighter Health Predictive Readiness Analytics, Joint Artificial Intelligence Center

"Dr. Tetteh, an accomplished surgeon, AI strategist, and public servant, takes readers on a journey into healthcare's future in *Smarter Healthcare with AI*. With compelling insights into the potential impact of AI on health and healthcare delivery, Dr. Tetteh outlines a visionary framework for bringing AI into healthcare. It is a must-read for all healthcare workers, technology enthusiasts, and policymakers, exploring how AI can democratize access to medical technologies and create a more efficient, patient-centric system."

—Andrew D. Plummer, MD, MPH
Captain (retired), US Public Health Service | Veteran and Founder, InnerLearn LLC

"Just as the US Navy advanced from dead reckoning to satellite navigation, Captain (Dr.) Hassan Tetteh plots a course through the waters of artificial intelligence in medicine. His new book, *Smarter Healthcare with AI*, proposes that AI models can elevate data to improve health and save lives. He expertly navigates the tides, winds, and currents of today's digital landscape by combining cutting-edge science with Hippocratic wisdom. Dr. Tetteh is taking the helm—*Smarter Healthcare with AI* is a guiding map for those of us ready to make the voyage."

—Jeff Plummer
Captain (retired), US Navy | Life Fellow, American College of Healthcare Executives | Former Navy senior executive to MHS Governance, Defense Health Agency | Former senior executive, Office of the Surgeon General, Navy Bureau of Medicine and Surgery

"Dr. Tetteh's approaches AI with surgeon-like precision coupled with humility and depth. His multimodal approach to dealing with this promising, contentious, and controversial issue is remarkable. He humanizes and personalizes the exploration and implications of AI with purpose, insight, and vision. He gives us the key to unlock and understand AI and its interface with health caring. His style is engaging, thoughtful and incisive."

—Dennis Robbins, PhD, MPH

Principal, Person Centric Solutions | Former National Fund for Medical Education Fellow at Harvard | Former Head of Joint Military Health Think Tank

"Dr. Hassan Tetteh brings his considerable experience as a military surgeon, author, strategist, and, importantly, humane and compassionate healer to the emerging field of AI. In his new book *Smarter Healthcare with AI: Harnessing Military Medicine to Revolutionize Healthcare for Everyone, Everywhere*, Dr. Tetteh draws from his diverse experience to envision a future that harnesses real world experience to articulate a way ahead for the complex tool of AI that is tempered by an understanding of the essential constraints that use this tool effectively. Anchored in a vision of Purpose, Personalization, Partnership, and Productivity and with the mindset of discipline, synthesis, creativity, respect, and ethics, Dr. Tetteh suggests tempering the raw technical power of AI with the human elements that support the philosophy he provides in these constructs. A worthwhile read to get oriented and a sound guide to the emerging impact of AI on healthcare practice and delivery."

—Keith L. Salzman, MD, MPH

Diplomate, Clinical Informatics, FAAFP | Colonel (retired), US Army | Salzman HCIT Consulting LLC

"Dr. Hassan Tetteh is a fervent advocate for healthcare, demonstrating his commitment by traveling globally to deliver organs to patients in need of transplants. His recognition of the transformative potential of AI in healthcare is unsurprising, given his vision for making high-quality, reliable healthcare more accessible. Dr. Tetteh's personal experiences with medical errors further fuel his drive to leverage AI for improved healthcare outcomes, a perspective he elaborates on in his book. By championing AI, he aims to inspire others to embrace this innovative approach for a better future in healthcare."

—Miles Smallhorne
University at Buffalo graduate student | Management Information Systems (2025)

"Hassan's many contributions to the fields of medicine, science, innovation, and the arts is a testament to his breadth of knowledge, commitment to patients, and strong desire to 'make the impossible, possible.' With every new challenge, Hassan leads with genuine empathy, selfless devotion, and an unyielding desire to improve the lives of everyone. He is fearless. His foray into the world of AI and health will no doubt push the boundaries as he works relentlessly to harness the power of AI for good. He is not on the vanguard—Hassan IS the vanguard."

—Robin Strongin
Board member, Lewy Body Dementia Resource Center

"Dr. Hassan Tetteh speaks to AI enthusiasts and skeptics. Drawing from his eclectic and impressive background as a US Navy cardiothoracic surgeon with combat experience, chief medical informatics officer, department of defense AI strategist, and scholar, Dr. Tetteh outlines the possibilities and benefits of leveraging AI and Military Medicine. This book is for healthcare providers who want to enhance their capability and productivity without compromising equitable, personalized, and ethical care. Dr. Tetteh demonstrates how every healthcare team member can leverage AI to promote health, prevent disease, enhance surgical techniques, and improve infectious disease management. Dr. Tetteh is an inspirational writer whose wisdom speaks to the heart and mind—this book will move you to action."

—Melissa Troncoso, PHD, FNP-C, CHWC
Captain, Nursing Corps, US Navy | Assistant clinical professor, Uniformed Services University of the Health Sciences

"In *Smarter Healthcare with AI*, Dr. Tetteh adeptly illustrates how AI, drawing from advancements in military medicine, can revolutionize healthcare delivery, making it more personalized, efficient, and equitable. Dr. Tetteh's pioneering VP4 Framework—purpose, personalization, partnership, and productivity—offers a visionary approach to integrating AI into health systems, ensuring that the benefits of technology are accessible to all.

His real-world examples and ethical considerations enrich the narrative, providing a clear and practical guide for healthcare professionals and policymakers eager to embrace the potential of AI. The book's emphasis on creating an inclusive data ecosystem that empowers individuals to take control of their health data is particularly inspiring and aligns with the evolving landscape of patient-centered care.

Smarter Healthcare with AI is a vital contribution to the field of healthcare and technology. It not only highlights the profound impact of AI but also sets a road map for future innovations. I am confident that this book will become an essential resource for anyone involved in the intersection of technology and medicine."

—John H. Stewart, IV, MD, MBA, FACS
Professor and chair of surgery, Morehouse School of Medicine | Oncology Programs

SMARTER HEALTHCARE
WITH AI

HASSAN A. TETTEH, MD

SMARTER HEALTHCARE
WITH AI•

HARNESSING MILITARY MEDICINE TO REVOLUTIONIZE HEALTHCARE FOR EVERYONE, EVERYWHERE

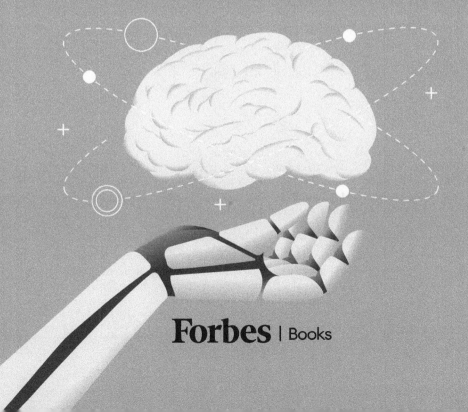

Forbes | Books

The opinions and assertions expressed herein are those of the author(s) and do not reflect the official policy or position of the Uniformed Services University of the Health Sciences or the Department of Defense.

Published by Forbes Books, Charleston, South Carolina.
An imprint of Advantage Media Group.

Forbes Books is a registered trademark, and the Forbes Books colophon is a trademark of Forbes Media, LLC.

Printed in the United States of America.

10 9 8 7 6 5 4 3 2 1

ISBN: 979-8-88750-481-0 (Hardcover)
ISBN: 979-8-88750-482-7 (eBook)

Library of Congress Control Number: 2024916192

Book design by Analisa Smith.
Author photo by Peter Cutts.

This custom publication is intended to provide accurate information and the opinions of the author in regard to the subject matter covered. It is sold with the understanding that the publisher, Forbes Books, is not engaged in rendering legal, financial, or professional services of any kind. If legal advice or other expert assistance is required, the reader is advised to seek the services of a competent professional.

Since 1917, Forbes has remained steadfast in its mission to serve as the defining voice of entrepreneurial capitalism. Forbes Books, launched in 2016 through a partnership with Advantage Media, furthers that aim by helping business and thought leaders bring their stories, passion, and knowledge to the forefront in custom books. Opinions expressed by Forbes Books authors are their own. To be considered for publication, please visit **books.Forbes.com**.

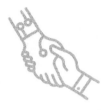

*To Edmund Emmanuel Tetteh, "My Wisdom,"
and Ella Bleue Tetteh, "My Inspiration"*

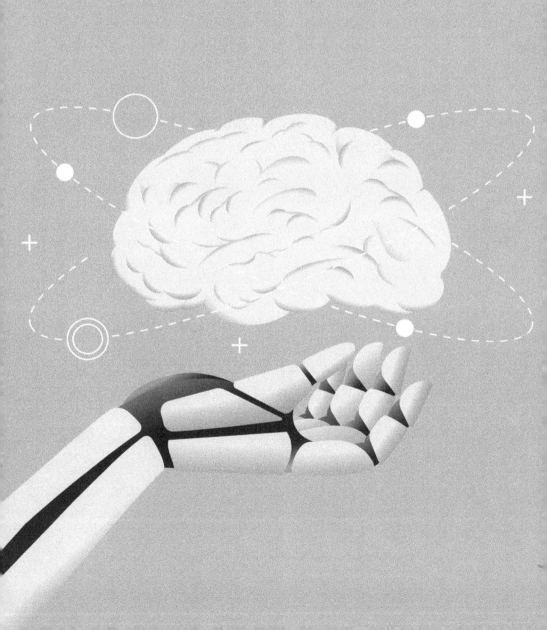

CONTENTS

FOREWORD

The day I embarked on writing this foreword was the same day Dr. Hassan Tetteh honored me by joining our executive leadership team at AI MINDSystems Foundation, where I serve as chief executive officer and cofounder. I'm proud that he is now our chief veterans' health officer, one of several esteemed cofounders, and the leader of our National HERO (Health Enhancing Resource Orchestration) initiative.

The National HERO cohort we seek to serve is composed of four groups: active duty service members, veterans of the United States Armed Forces, all first responders, and the immediate families of these groups, including their children. Dr. Tetteh's twenty-five years of service in the United States Navy, his extensive clinical experience spanning cardiac and thoracic surgery with a specialization in heart and lung transplantology and informatics broadly, and his very unique experiences in health AI within the Department of Defense are all part of what makes Dr. Tetteh a remarkable fit to lead the National HERO initiative—but it is more than these things. By reading *Smarter Healthcare with AI*, you will encounter Dr. Tetteh's compassion, empathy, wisdom, powerful conviction, and clear vision for elevating human potentials and human experiences through ethical AI.

The National HERO initiative will launch two interdependent programs. One is to create a number of WISDOM (Worldwide Informatics System and Data Ontology Matrix) Networks—a new class of replicable utility for multiparty ethical AI and collaborative computing. In WISDOM Networks, the source data of participating enterprises in the public and private sector remain decentralized. Through the incorporation of blockchain and multiple privacy-enhancing technologies, trusted and verifiable multiparty data analytics and ethical AI can be administered, orchestrated, and operated in a verifiably compliant, ethically intentional, transparent, accountable framework. Over time, we believe this framework will rebuild broken trust in our social systems, institutions, and digital experiences as it scales.

WISDOM Networks will be governed in AI MINDSystems Foundation's new construct for public-private-*person* partnerships (P^4). This is the first approach to formally include individuals, families, and communities in public-private partnerships legally, financially, operationally, and technologically. This is part of our broader P^4 Framework for Systemic Innovation™ to bring about a trusted data ecosystem, a financially just and inclusive data economy, and ethical AI. This next generation of AI will be truly person centered and literally person sovereign and will interact with an endless array of other AIs operated by enterprises and governments. Many of the AI models trained within the ecosystem will learn exclusively from the person's own data that has been brought under their direct custody. These self-sovereign AIs—we call them "Trusted Agents"—will be administered and hosted in an infrastructure controlled solely by the person and operated under a business model that mitigates potential conflicts of interest with the person.

Our approach is very consistent with Dr. Tetteh's idea as reflected in this book, especially by his VP4 AI Framework: purpose, personalization, partnership, and productivity. (We independently arrived at names that involved "P4" for our complementary ideas—working together was clearly meant to be!)

This person-centered strategy that we're talking about facilitates the creation of decentralized yet massively multimodal AI—both for model training and at runtime. By multimodal, I mean many very diverse data domains, each with distinct data features, about a common data subject. For example, this could be multiple silos of EHR data from various providers where you have received care; insurance claims data from multiple health plans in which you've been a member; pharmacy data where you've had prescriptions filled; Internet-of-Things data from many devices, social media data, and location data; and especially your full-sequence human genome and sixteen other types of very sensitive biometric data we believe only you should control. This kind of data, especially when combined with many other data domains about you, requires advanced security and privacy that are not yet available or understandable to most people.

While every health-related enterprise, both in the public and private sectors, wishes to use AI to improve patient outcomes and experiences, data acquisition and ethical AI and data governance remain enormous challenges as of the publication of this book. There is no way that healthcare provider organizations can assemble very many full-context, identified, and fully verifiable data domains about an individual patient or research subject in all needed contexts of verification. The best they can do is to make probabilistic guesses through the use of de-identified data purchased from various data brokers in order to add data domains and dimensionality to the data they originated in-house.

Furthermore, while there is controversy on this point, generally, these organizations need to have consent to use this data they originated for secondary purposes—such as to train AI models. Today, typical data use—related consents are not suited to the realities of what's now needed for ethical AI and data governance in healthcare and life sciences. Instead, the future state of AI-related consents and authorizations need to be

1. part of multiparty workflows involving both the data subject and authorized actors within a given institution;

2. granular to enable selective disclosure;

3. context sensitive to ensure the consent is associated with a clearly communicated purpose by a known set of parties;

4. time bound such that indefinite data use doesn't occur unless expressly permitted;

5. dynamic as the circumstances of an original consent may change, and the data subject's decisions may change accordingly;

6. cryptographically and forensically verifiable on demand by any regulator, institutional review board, or compliance office; and

7. easily revokable within an easy-to-understand process describing what is and isn't possible to achieve in the event a consent is withdrawn after a model is already in production.

Ongoing AI-related legal challenges will slow AI's extraordinary potential for good until we have trusted methods obtaining "AI-appropriate" data use consents from data subjects with the characteristics described above. Furthermore, that is all related to consent for model *training*—model *usage* "on" a patient, member, or social services recipient brings yet another set of important considerations with corresponding new legislation, regulation, and policy in the United States and jurisdictions around the world.

The data acquisition approach that was used historically to train many of the AI models that have already been deployed to production in healthcare contexts—often as embedded components of larger and more complex workflow or clinical decision support systems or as tools regulated as software as a medical device, such as digital diagnostics and digital therapeutics—has a series of problems. I mention two of them relevant to this book and to my shared work with Dr. Tetteh.

First, huge swaths of humanity with mental and physical health problems—estimated by the World Bank in 2024 to exceed 1.5 billion people—are not *patients* at all because they have literally no access to care. Data about them simply isn't in the health system, so it can't have informed training AI models for use in healthcare settings or been included in clinical research participant recruitment for new vaccines, drugs, medical devices, and digital interventions.

In the United States, a huge swath of patients doesn't consistently receive evidence-based, equitable, accessible, and affordable care. What data exists about this very large group of patients is sparse and spotty—not at all like what it would be were those same patients to have been in consistent and appropriate preventative care and treatment protocols.

Second, in the United States, many data modalities are extremely relevant to mental and physical health, but they are not originated in a healthcare context by HIPAA-covered entities. Thus, they are not regulated as "protected health information" (PHI) by the US Department of Health and Human Services. This includes a wide range of data potentially impactful in addressing environmental and social determinants of health and achieving the vision of precision health for us all. Because it isn't PHI under the law, this data is not subject to the anti-information blocking provisions enabling portability of a subset of PHI under the 21st Century Cures Act. Personal data access and portability is a major missing piece from United States Federal Trade Commission regulated data. Personal data is originated in all of our walks of life, in the enormous and growing volume of data we each generate every single day simply by living in modernity. All of our digital experiences, location data, financial data, social data, every transaction we make, every click on every site on every app, every device, every interaction—it is all presently being collected, used, and often monetized in de-identified form in transactions that technically remain legal but are unknown to most people. When large data monetization transactions have been picked up in the press, these transactions have often been met with shock and anger by the patients and customers of the organizations selling the data. Many feel that if data about us is being monetized—regardless of whether it is de-identified—we should be part of that decision-making and not be excluded in that economic value chain. This includes the leaders at AI MINDSystems Foundation.

When we begin to train AI models to learn and optimize for the person across all of those data modalities under their own custody, with complete and verifiable privacy preservation, we think the impact on the person has the potential to be absolutely radical. There are tens of thousands of continuously changing variables in an individual person's life that could affect their well-being, prosperity, and goal achievement. We mean people's own personal aims—not the aims of the companies they choose to do business with, their health system, their health insurance company, their employer, or their government. That can only happen through self-sovereign AIs interacting with AIs operated by all of these parties external to us, operating for us, solely on our behalf, and verifiably absent any conflict of interest. Dr. Tetteh's vision and articulation—and his VP4 framework—will all be very important contributions to the realization of this vision.

The VP4 framework is a perfect mapping of the capabilities and resources we hope to bring to the world in our envisioned new data economy and trusted data ecosystem. This new system and social structure will enable individuals, families, communities, and affinity groups to achieve and protect data sovereignty and privacy and the significant empowerment this can unlock. Your Trusted Agents, interacting with and continuously optimizing in your personal interest and automating on your behalf, can nearly instantaneously process far more discrete details than any naturally intelligent human being could ever manually process and act upon. Your personal, self-sovereign digital twin will continuously grow more powerfully predictive and able to determine methods to aid your total well-being according to what is meaningful and most important to you.

Our work at the AI MINDSystems Foundation is an extension and an operationalization of Dr. Tetteh's vision for how these data partnerships with patients can work. In order to create this new framework, to begin a deep structural and systemic intervention, it is necessary to create a flywheel effect. We have to start a *virtuous* cycle that can reverse the *vicious* cycles that have been playing out, resulting in ever-increasing per capita healthcare expenditures and worsening health equity and population health outcomes. Under Dr. Tetteh's incredible leadership, the AI MINDSystems Foundation's National HERO Initiative will achieve this immensely important goal. Dr. Tetteh's method for doing this is charted in this book, *Smarter Healthcare with AI*.

—HEATHER LEIGH FLANNERY
Chief Executive Officer and Cofounder
AI MINDSystems Foundation and Trusted Data Ecosystem

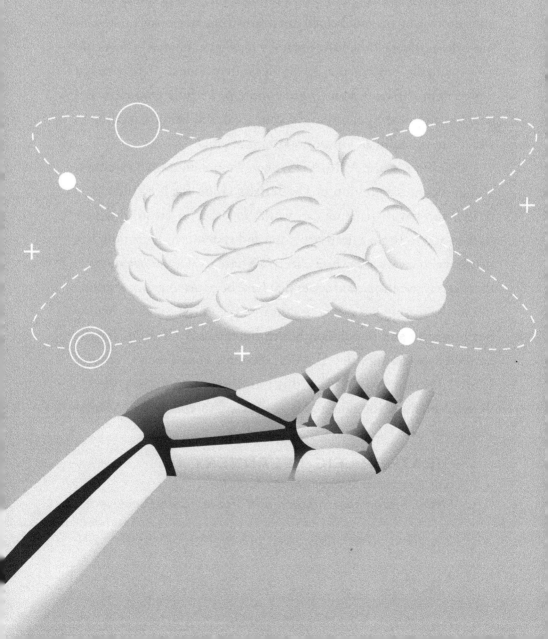

INTRODUCTION

" How do we prepare for the future with AI?" This is a question many are asking and one I'm always excited to answer. Why? Because I believe AI will usher us into the next best level of healthcare.

Even the most disciplined physicians can become overwhelmed in today's infinitely complex healthcare world. Synthesizing information, making the right connections to create optimal treatment plans, and respecting the differences between individual patients and their medical needs are all big asks. They must do all of this while handling each case ethically and with the intention of building upon medical knowledge and practice. AI brings hope to these physicians.

Howard Gardner, one of my former professors and a scholar, described and popularized the concept of multiple intelligences in his book *Five Minds for the Future*. I have clung to his work, and it has proven itself over all these decades. Gardner's five minds provide a framework for being successful and ushering AI into the realm of healthcare. These five minds are as follows:

1. **A disciplined mind.** This mind has a deep understanding of three classical principles: truth, beauty, and goodness, based on the mastery of the major disciplines that we have created over the centuries.

2. **A synthesizing mind.** This mind assembles and synthesizes information we gather from the internet and beyond. Knowledge is only potential power. It's how you apply that knowledge that makes it actionable.

3. **A creative mind.** This mind makes connections, asks and answers questions that have not been asked, and creates art, music, and all the achievements that define humankind. Responses generated from creative prompts on ChatGPT especially represent this mind through large language models trained on the expanse of human knowledge.

4. **A respectful mind.** This mind is cognizant and respectful of the differences in individuals. We can see across the world that when people don't respect differences or try to crush or suppress them, the result is tumult, animosity, wars, and conflict.

5. **An ethical mind.** This mind embraces ethical values and fulfills the obligation to pass one's craft to the next generation.

AI applications and solutions have been game changers, and they are now setting the foundation for the future of healthcare delivery. Artificial intelligence (AI) is fundamentally evolving the delivery of healthcare for people around the world. The potential for AI tools to impact healthcare even more in the coming years presents opportunities and challenges as we create safe, equitable, and effective solutions.

My first book, *Gifts of the Heart*, was recently released as a second edition on its tenth anniversary. This novel parallels my experience as a medical officer in the deserts of Afghanistan during Operation Enduring Freedom. The subsequent *The Art of Human Care* series has addressed many facets of the healthcare world through my philosophy of purpose, personalization, and partnerships. These books explore not only my experiences as a thoracic surgeon doing heart and lung transplants but also the history of medicine, healthcare applications in the military, the COVID-19 pandemic, *LIFE: Love in Full Effect*, and AI.

As a heart and lung surgeon in the military for twenty-five years, I spent five of those years working with AI applications focused on medical care. In my final years of service with the US Navy before my retirement in 2023, I served as an AI strategist in the Department of Defense (DoD). Here, I found myself on the front lines of the changing landscape of healthcare delivery with AI at the epicenter.

Historically, the military has been at the forefront of healthcare. War brings injury and disease. Soldiers must be healed so they can continue the good fight and return home to their families. Military medicine is already harnessing the power of AI, making advances that have made the impossible possible and evolved the art of healing around the world.

With AI, military medicine has harnessed massive amounts of data with incredible computing power to manage electronic health records (EHRs) with advanced machine learning algorithms. Government and commercial investments have converged to create unprecedented AI opportunities to change the delivery of healthcare. Providers who don't want to get on board will be forced to. Why? Because their patients will be looking for answers. AI will be the norm and not the exception at some point—not too far off.

But there's a chasm right now, and it's time to bridge it.

While I have been a Forbes Technology Council member for years, this is my first opportunity to work with Forbes Books, for which I am grateful. This volume will inspire readers to build that bridge with five spans: discipline, synthesis, creativity, respect, and ethics.

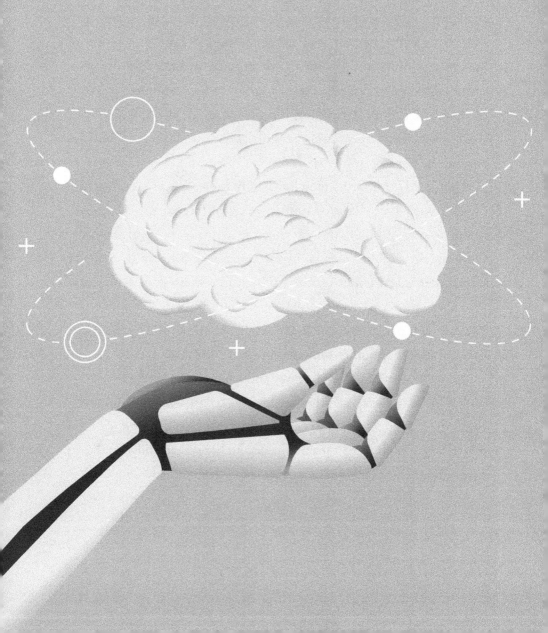

CHAPTER 1

THEY CALL ME
THE "UNICORN"

AI is fundamentally evolving the delivery of healthcare for people around the world. Yet the potential for AI tools to impact healthcare in the coming years presents opportunities and challenges to ensure these solutions will be safe, equitable, and effective.

So how did a heart and lung surgeon like me end up leading the charge for implementing AI in healthcare? Well, I spent twenty-five years of my career with the US Navy, the last decade of which I led enterprise technology implementation as the chief medical informatics officer for the US Navy and as the Warfighter Health Mission chief for the DoD Joint Artificial Intelligence Center (JAIC).

The JAIC's other divisions and teams worked to leverage AI to ensure that America's combat operations lead and remain at the cutting edge of machine learning in troop readiness, cybersecurity, joint maneuvers, and lethality. My team's task was to leverage and implement AI solutions to improve warfighter health.

My national security and military history studies at the National War College informed my work. I knew the military had led the charge in medical breakthroughs that ultimately improved healthcare for civilian populations throughout history—more about that in chapter 2. From my prior academic studies of clinical informatics at Stanford University, Harvard Kennedy School, and Johns Hopkins Carey Business School, I concluded AI was a tool that could improve the delivery of healthcare and make care more personalized.

Make the Impossible Possible and Change Healing around the World

My experience at the JAIC allowed me to apply theory and accumulated knowledge to synthesize my ideas into a concrete reality. I knew that if our military harnessed the power of AI for warfighter health, our advances would begin to make the impossible possible and change healing around the world.

Lieutenant General John "Jack" N. T. Shanahan, a three-star United States Air Force retiree, was appointed as the first director of the DoD JAIC. His appointment was based on his previous work with Project Maven, the Pentagon's leading AI program, which focused on utilizing AI computer vision for security and intelligence purposes. Established in 2018, the JAIC aimed to leverage the transformative potential of AI to enhance the United States' national security.

National security is based on a strong military, and the health of our forces and warfighter health emerged as one of the JAIC's spheres of interest. I had the luck and serendipity of being recruited to lead the new warfighter health division of the JAIC. After spending his first fifteen years in fighter aviation, beginning with the F-4 and then the F-15E, General Shanahan was assigned six different and very diverse commands, starting with an intelligence group squadron of a hundred people and ending with a twenty-seven-thousand-person air force command.

Then he arrived at the JAIC. Since he led and established the JAIC, I'll let him tell this part of the story.

The JAIC was the department's first foray into AI in everything beyond intelligence, including medicine. We would not have embarked on medical projects without a medical expert. That's why Hassan was so important given his background and interest in AI.

We would not have taken on warfighter health had we not had someone like Dr. Tetteh come on board. Hassan, he's one of a kind. He's sweet, as the Latin term *suavis* is defined: pleasant, inviting, kind, agreeable, delightful. He's generous. He was an active cardiothoracic surgeon. He went to the National War College. He's interested in AI—he actually wrote his War College thesis on how AI can revolutionize healthcare. This is something he was passionate about.

I didn't know him. I didn't know how to find somebody with his background. But here he was, a senior officer in the Navy. According to the *Oxford Dictionary*, a unicorn can be defined as "something that is highly desirable but difficult to find or obtain." Hassan was our unicorn.

In AI, you have two camps. You have people who are very theoretical about AI and love talking about the theory of what AI can do and what it can't do. Then you have a technology community that dives in and develops these technologies without really considering the long-term societal effects. Hassan understood.

He didn't come in as an AI expert but knew enough about it. He could write about AI and healthcare all day long. But he didn't just write about it. He came in, and I put him in charge of our Warfighter Health Initiative. He jumped in and figured out how to start these projects and how to find talent with a medical background who could help him. He crossed between these two worlds of the theoretical and the practical—and you just do not find a person who can do that very often.

Standing up this organization was a very steep hill to climb. But here comes somebody who's got it all. I'll never forget him taking several of us over to watch open-heart surgery at one of the local hospitals—an amazing, amazing experience—and, during the surgery, he was pointing out where AI could have helped.

So I designated Hassan to run our Warfighter Health Mission initiative. One of the first things we did was work with the Joint Pathology Center. We worked with fifty million physical slides with pathology samples, everything from viruses to tissue. First, they needed to be digitized. They were old-fashioned slides sitting in the Joint Pathology Center. It's a monumental undertaking to digitize. Once it's done, however, they can be used for all sorts of research purposes. The hope was to use AI, machine learning, or deep learning to go through these samples and find patterns that could predict what might happen in the future.

I remember they had COVID-19 samples from the late '60s and early '70s, early versions of COVID-19. It struck all of us. If these had been digitized and analyzed with AI, maybe we could have gotten to a COVID-19 vaccine even faster than we did. The idea of being a little more predictive about what might be coming down the road is incredibly powerful. Hassan embarked on that and made a lot of progress.

We also had a project that addressed suicide and suicidal ideations by military members. It allowed us to look at past evidence and data and make it a little easier for commanders to predict when a particular service member might be close to suicidal ideation. We were very careful about how we used the data, but suicide causes a great deal of tragedy, turmoil, and turbulence in the military. One individual suicide is devastating to families, the health of an organization, and warfighting readiness.

Another area we studied was better battlefield treatment. We looked at how quickly a service member was triaged and treated when wounded. We looked for opportunities to use AI to accelerate the process, for example, by sending a drone in with blood supply.

There was no shortage of issues to work on. During the pandemic, we started Project Salus, an AI tool that helped the National Guard analyze critical supply-chain data to predict COVID-19 hot spots and related logistics issues before they happened.

We also looked at how AI could improve healthcare through preventive and predictive medicine, which directly and immediately impacts warfighter readiness. The healthier the force and the healthier the families of the service members, the better we'll do as a warfighting force.

The idea of preventive healthcare is enormously important. Using AI, we're starting to find indicators of problems before they have blossomed into full-blown problems. It's an endless opportunity that hasn't moved as quickly as any of us would like. However, there are encouraging signs that this is something the government realizes could be very important.

AI has the potential to help our military better address the healthcare needs of those serving our country on active duty and after they are discharged as veterans. An awful lot happens during the transition from active duty to becoming veterans that could be helped by AI, including being evaluated for disabilities.

Look at the magnitude of this in the veterans' programs alone. In 2022 the United States spent more than $272 billion on the disability program and medical care for veterans. We spent another $55.8 billion on active duty members, retired members, and family members under the Military Health System. Those numbers are staggering. It could make an incredible difference if we can find a way to use AI to help chip away at those dollars.

AI developments made by the military will also advance healthcare in the civilian population. What makes AI so interesting is something that we call "dual use." In the military we're used to dealing with technologies that were developed by companies that work for the military. These tend to be warfighting systems built for the military, by the military, and with the military. AI has this dual-use capability in that, for the most part, it has been coming out of commercial industry. There's great research going on in the military on AI, but the day-to-day applications that are making the most difference right now are coming from the commercial sector.

If I were to look at medicine, healthcare, and warfighter health, AI is one area that equally applies to the military and the civilian community. So what the civilian world is doing with AI will help the military, and what the military is working on with AI could help the civilian community. There are countless opportunities to work side by side.

Some companies are reluctant to work with the DoD on warfighting systems for moral and ethical reasons. For example, they may be concerned about lethal autonomous weapons systems. When it comes to healthcare, I don't see any of those concerns. In fact, it's just the opposite. People understand that this is one area that everybody in the United States can fully embrace—the military's use of AI for healthcare. Lines that are starkly drawn when discussing warfighting systems dissolve when we look at healthcare because everybody realizes how important it is to our well-being, national security, health, and financial standing.

Electronic medical records are another area where AI can be of tremendous help. There are privacy concerns, as is expected when medical records are involved. However, AI applications can rapidly transition between the civilian and military populations as service members retire and become civilians or retirees. AI-enhanced electronic medical records can also benefit huge swaths of the civilian population, bringing the costs of hospitals and healthcare down.

The idea of people being the center of attention—there is an unfortunate tendency today to focus on technology at the expense of the human. I call it technological determinism:

"Just leave us alone in Silicon Valley, and we'll figure it out, and all will be right with the world."

I don't accept that because it forgets that people are the recipients of this technology. People need a voice, and they need to feel that whatever this technology is, however advanced it may be, doesn't completely remove a human from the equation.

Anybody who's actually done AI in the production process will say it is the combination of a human and a smart machine working together. Humans do things that only humans can do, still to this day, for a long time to come. Deductive reasoning, inductive reasoning, abductive reasoning, context, putting yourself in a patient's shoes—a machine has no concept of what that even means.

Machines do this: they process data. They're intelligent. AI can improve the entire DoD, from undersea to outer space and everything in between. And that includes VA evaluation and disability assessment. There are just so many different places where AI could be used.

At the JAIC, Hassan brought such an interesting background to the table. He's enthusiastic. He's a great speaker. He's always out and about. There's just nobody else like him. That's why I called him a unicorn. I stand by that today because I still don't think there's anybody quite like him out there.

Humble Beginnings

Both General Shanahan and I have since retired from our careers with the military and our work with the JAIC. But we haven't retired from being active proponents of using AI to deliver higher-quality healthcare to both the military and civilian world. My military career began in 1998 when I raised my hand to support and defend the Constitution of the United States by accepting a commission in the United States Navy. Over my years of service, Dr. Michael Malanoski was perhaps one of the most consequential individuals in my military career. Dr. Malanoski currently serves as the deputy director of the Defense Health Agency (DHA). The DHA is a joint, integrated combat support agency that enables medical services for the Army, Navy, and Air Force "to provide a medically ready force and ready medical force" in both peacetime and wartime.

When I first met Dr. Malanoski in 2003, he was still in uniform and serving as the Navy's general surgery specialty leader. He was responsible for assigning surgeons throughout the world where they were most needed. Dr. Malanoski gave me my first assignment as the ship's surgeon on the USS *Carl Vinson*.

I recall the moment vividly. Dr. Malanoski collected a group of us—all new surgeons—just as our officer indoctrination program was coming to an end. Most of my colleagues, all the other doctors, nurses, and lawyers from the Judge Advocate General's Corps were heading off to nice, cushy assignments at hospitals and in clinics. Dr. Malanoski looked at my name tag and said, "Oh, you, Tetteh. That's right. I just changed your orders. You're not going to the ship that is docked there on the pier. I'm going to send you on the *Carl Vinson*."

I said, "Okay, sir."

I immediately went to my chief petty officer and said, "Hey, they just changed my orders. I'm going to the *Vinson*. Where is that?"

My chief answered, "That's one of the aircraft carriers, and she is deployed."

So I asked, "Oh, do I report to the duty station, hang out, and wait for the ship to return?"

My chief replied, "Well, no, no. It doesn't work like that, sir. You'll get on a plane, and they'll fly you out."

Within a few days of that fateful first meeting with Dr. Malanoski, I flew over the vast Pacific Ocean thousands of feet in the air and appreciated the USS *Carl Vinson* (CVN-70) from far above. She looked like a postage stamp in the middle of the ocean—and I would soon land on her and call her home. This would be my first real military assignment. I was fresh out of residency, the only surgeon on an aircraft carrier with over six thousand men and women who had all raised their hands to serve.

Now the *Vinson* was coming back from a deployment. The crew had been out to sea for many, many months. And I was the brand-new surgeon among a seasoned and salty medical team. Soon after my arrival, we all met to review the statistics of the many cases treated during the deployment. We had this many appendicitis cases. We had this many fractures. We had this many infections. When it was reported that we had thirteen pregnancies, I turned to my senior medical officer, Dr. Danny Holman. In front of the entire medical team, who were just being introduced to me, their brand-new surgeon, I asked, "Sir, how does that happen?"

Dr. Holman turned to the rest of the medical team and said, "Okay, medical, let's tell the surgeon how babies are made."

I spent twenty-two months on that ship—nineteen of them in deep blue water operations. This gave me and my colleagues the unique distinction of being able to scrape salt off our shoulders because we'd spent so much time out at sea. That experience also helped me understand the three underlying tenets of the US Navy: honor, courage, and commitment.

Subsequent assignments with the US Navy took me to medical-surgical tents in the deserts of Afghanistan, the great African continent amid the Ebola epidemic, the Middle East, Europe, and the South Pacific. I literally went around the world on a ship. And in the desert, with bombs and missiles flying overhead, we took care of blown-up Marines.

Indeed, the many experiences I had in the military were unique. However, I am convinced my background and these collective experiences, as General Shanahan and others observed, contributed to my "unicorn" moniker. When I was in the tents in Afghanistan with bombs flying overhead, when I heard that aircraft carriers were the most dangerous places on earth, or when they told me, "You better be careful here in Africa," I would always say to myself, "Yeah, but this is not Broadway Junction. None of these experiences have anything on Broadway Junction. It's not that bad."

Nothing compared to the fear I felt growing up in the 1980s and 1990s in Brooklyn, New York, on the subway platform of the A train at Broadway Junction. Overcoming that fear and surviving commuting to school every day created resolve and tenacity. My Brooklyn experience, those formative years raised as the son of West African immigrant parents, my work as a heart surgeon, and years of military service all prepared me for the great task of this moment—a calling to deliver smarter healthcare with AI.

From the A Train to the AI Team

Weeks before my retirement, a young man saw my uniform hanging up. He looked at it and said, "Hey, you're in the Navy. Thank you for your service." Having heard this statement many times, I calmly responded, "Thank you for saying that."

He pushed back, saying, "No, no, no. I really mean *thank you* for your service. I'm not from this country. Thank you for your service because you're doing the things I don't want to do to improve America and the world. But more importantly, because in my country, it's not like it is in America. So I'm thanking you because you're doing things I don't want to do. You're doing what makes America, America."

The young man was from Haiti, and his perspective at that moment, just before I transitioned to civilian life, was poignant. He was happy to be living in America and saw my service as a reason America was desirable. Indeed, I recognized his gratitude for living in America. It was similar to the feelings of hope, promise, and aspiration my immigrant parents espoused for being citizens of America.

This brief encounter caused me to reflect. I began to appreciate the service concept and theme of duty in a different way. Machiavelli once said, "If you have a good idea, you better have an army." If you have a good idea, like the one that's embodied in the principles of the preamble of the US Constitution, that makes this country better than any other country on the planet despite its quirks, despite its problems, despite its issues, then you not only better have an army, but you also better have a navy, a marine corps, an air force, a coast guard, and a space force. You better have leading-edge healthcare to keep those organizations operating at top efficiency.

We must provide the best care available for medical and behavioral health issues, whether for warfighters or the civilian population they are sworn to protect. We need to advance not only new surgical techniques, vaccine developments, and medication innovations but also the use of AI. The current healthcare system is bogged down by its own immensity, the number of records, an overburdened workforce, and a complex reimbursement system.

In the hands of caring physicians and nurses, AI can usher the "personal" back into medicine. In the databases of vast healthcare systems and insurance providers, AI can speed diagnoses, help tailor treatment plans, and reduce costs in billing, filing claims, and processing payments. In the hands of the people—literally as an app on their phones—AI can help individuals monitor their own conditions and encourage lifestyle choices that promote health.

People have asked me what my plans are now that I've retired from the Navy. And I always tell them I will commit myself to inspiring, healing, teaching, leading, and serving. Most importantly, I will work every day to create the greatest good for humankind.

When I went to the War College, I was the only physician in my class of two hundred warfighters—future classmates who would be generals, admirals, and great military minds. Many of those warfighters were smart, talented cyber and intelligence community leaders who had been looking at intel and data. My conversations with them inspired me to write my master's thesis about how AI could enhance military medicine. That thesis, *AI and Military Medicine: Strategic Application of the Technology of Our Era*, was the document that caught the attention of the people building a new team at the DoD dedicated to leveraging AI: the JAIC. That team included General Shanahan.

However, during my twenty-five years with the Navy, I also served as an associate professor of surgery at the Uniformed Services University of the Health Sciences and adjunct faculty at Howard University College of Medicine. At the "heart" of it all, I am a physician and surgeon. In this role, and in working to balance clinical medicine with administrative responsibilities and the burgeoning field of AI, I found myself increasingly attracted to the world of heart and lung transplant, a passion I developed during training at the University of Minnesota. I eventually founded and led a Specialized

Thoracic Adapted Recovery (STAR) team in Washington, DC, and did research in organ transplantation to expand donation and save lives. For over fifteen years, we recovered heart and lung organs across the country and delivered them to waiting recipients wherever they were hospitalized. Our team recovered more than a thousand hearts and lungs.

My Calling, My Purpose

Both of my parents have passed away. Two West African immigrants, my mother and father believed strongly in the American Dream, and their particular American Dream was that their son would become a doctor. They both must be credited for creating an environment for success and influencing my motivation to pursue medicine as a career. A second motivator was my own near-death experience as a college student.

As a premed student in college, I interviewed at Johns Hopkins Medical School under an early decision program. I was beyond excited. After my interview, I knew I was destined to become a doctor. I returned to my small college in upstate New York to await the official news of my acceptance. Over the ensuing days, I became very ill with fever, chills, and the worst headache and neck pain of my life. I visited our college infirmary, was diagnosed (incorrectly) with gastroenteritis, prescribed penicillin tablets, and instructed to stay in bed and drink plenty of fluids.

My condition worsened. On a Friday night, I was alone in my dorm room and unable to call for help. Thankfully, two worried fraternity brothers entered my room to check on me. When they found me, I was lethargic and barely responsive. They rushed me to the local hospital emergency room. I recall bright lights and masked people hovering over me, sternal rubs, and being told to hold still because a needle was going into my back. The doctor said to me that I had a severe infection and could die.

I was a patient.

Many people experience being a patient in their lives but not always to this extreme. You are truly a patient when you are stripped of your clothes, wear the hospital-issued gown in humiliation, can no longer do anything for yourself, and have no idea what is going on. That happened to me. I did not understand what was happening. I was uncertain, anxious, and scared. I thought I was going to die.

Fortunately, my healing mind took over and did what medicine alone could not have done. Engendered by my recent interview for medical school, my spirited soul believed I was destined to become a healer.

In the days before my release from my weeks-long hospitalization, the attending emergency department doctor, Dr. Kevin McCullom, who'd taken care of me the day I was admitted, visited me. My friends had told him that I wanted to be a doctor.

Dr. McCullom presented me with a copy of *Harrison's Principles of Internal Medicine*. He showed me what kind of infection I had: bacterial meningitis. Together, we read about how serious the condition was and how it could have taken my life. He also told me that he had a test for me since I wanted to be a doctor. He proceeded to ask me, "What is two plus two?" I answered, "Four." He chuckled and said, "You will make a great doctor."

Decades have passed, yet I remember that ordeal as if it were yesterday. I also remember Dr. McCullom with gratitude for the great care he took to heal me. He helped me realize my purpose. That purpose not only spared a kid from Brooklyn from deadly meningitis but also inspired him to become a doctor who would, in time, be invited by other physicians to talk about human care.

My experience as an intensive care unit patient also taught me about empathy and what it feels like to be a patient. The average physician has approximately eighty thousand to one hundred thousand patient encounters over a typical career. Dr. McCullom potentially has one hundred thousand stories similar to mine that demonstrate the positive impact their encounter with him had on their lives.

Even brief encounters that seem inconsequential at the time can significantly impact a patient's life. In my comparatively short career, I've had the opportunity to help patients discover their purpose with the smallest effort. Through experiences like these and years of clinical experience, I've learned that one does not have to cure in order to heal. I realize that the work physicians do in this great profession gives them an incredible power, an amazing gift, to impact the lives of others in many meaningful ways. During their routine encounters, they may never fully appreciate the magnitude of that impact.

The Art of Human Care

Restoring health is an awesome purpose.

This purpose also inspired me to write my book series, *The Art of Human Care*. Purpose, personalization, and partnerships are the three fundamental pillars of *The Art of Human Care*. I've seen firsthand, and over the arc of history, how tools we've created as innovative humans have made healthcare better and pose a huge opportunity to improve healthcare overall. AI is our tool today.

The National Academy of Medicine (NAM), through the work of its members, research, studies, and influence, has changed the paradigm of practice and how healthcare is delivered. The NAM is now looking ahead at the next five years of healthcare. Front and center is AI. AI can help everyone involved in delivering healthcare, whether in a Mobile Army Surgical Hospital (MASH) tent in some forlorn desert or a high-tech operating suite in New York City. AI can streamline data to go beyond the law of averages to pinpoint an exact, highly personalized diagnosis for individual patients. AI can go beyond delivering a general message about diet, exercise, and healthy lifestyle choices to predicting exact health issues for individuals so they can be better-informed partners in their prevention.

Bringing AI into healthcare is about doctors and nurses caring for patients—human beings and their loved ones. AI is not the force ushering in a dystopian future. AI is the hope for an evolution of healthcare innovations that bring medical science back to its roots.

As General Shanahan mentioned, "A unicorn can be defined as 'something highly desirable but difficult to find or obtain.'" Good healthcare is like a unicorn for many in our communities today. It's highly desirable but difficult to obtain. I believe AI can help change that.

Into whatever houses I enter, I will go into them for the benefit of the sick.

—HIPPOCRATES

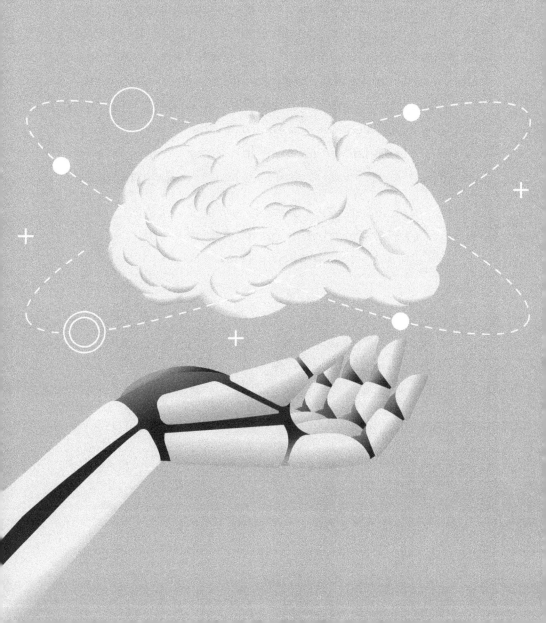

CHAPTER 2

THE MILITARY AND MEDICINE—THE HISTORY

It is not the strongest of the species that survive, nor the most intelligent, but the one most responsive to change.

—CHARLES DARWIN

W hen I talk about AI, I like to compare it to electricity. In the late nineteenth century, the electric light began transforming households, businesses, schools, hospitals—and the military. AI is the general-purpose technology of our era. The military has been among the early adopters of AI. I predict that it will also lead the charge when it comes to AI-enhanced healthcare delivery and healthcare systems management.

Indeed, the military is already using AI technology in healthcare. From augmented reality microscopes (ARM) to robotic process automation (RPA) for medical administrative tasks, AI is already impacting the landscape of the military's healthcare delivery and shaping its healthcare future. AI can help us understand disease in service members at a fundamentally better level and facilitate treatment to help wounded and sick service members more efficiently. As history has illustrated time and again, the revolutionary advances in medicine we enjoy have often originated with innovations in the military.

In 2016 I was selected to be the command surgeon at the National Defense University. Not only was I the first African American to be appointed to the role, but I was also the first naval officer selected to serve in the role after many years of being filled by an Army or Air Force officer. This background is significant and created a unique opportunity for the following two years to be very consequential for my work in AI.

Before my assignment at the National Defense University, I had the advantage of attending the Harvard Kennedy School of Government from 2008 to 2009. While there, I focused my studies on health policy, concentrating on health information technology. My experience at the Kennedy School was significant because I met and worked with incredible professors and was exposed to the power of independent study through a dynamic curriculum that was student centered and flexible.

During my tenure at the Kennedy School, I petitioned for an independent study project with Prof. Linda Bilmes, budgeting and finance instructor and coauthor with Joseph Stiglitz of *The Three Trillion Dollar War: The True Cost of the Iraq Conflict*. Professor Bilmes introduced me to leaders at the Veterans Affairs Administration (VA), including W. Scott Gould, former chief operating officer for the VA. With my interest in economics, health policy, and health information technology, we planned a study comparing the Armed Forces Health Longitudinal Technology Application (AHLTA) and Veterans Health Information Systems and Technology Architecture (VISTA) EHR platforms. My thesis paper eventually became a publication in *Military Medicine* titled, "Achieving Nirvana through an Electronic Medical Record System: A Military Surgeon's Perspective."

In my subsequent graduate work at Johns Hopkins Carey School of Business, while pursuing my MBA in Medical Services Management, I again concentrated on health information technology. I took advantage of another independent study opportunity. At Hopkins, my research study project focused on applying health technology to improve healthcare delivery. I coined the C.A.R.E. paradigm, which highlighted the collection, analysis, review, and evaluation of health data to improve health outcomes.

To capstone both respective graduate school studies at Harvard and Johns Hopkins, I was selected to be a Robert Wood Johnson Health Policy Fellow. I was fortunate to be assigned to the Congressional Budget Office (CBO) in the Health Analysis Division. My work at the CBO proved consequential because I learned about modeling and Bayesian statistics and was tasked with several projects to inform Congress of the budget option recommendations provided to save money in Medicare and Medicaid.

These historic experiences gave me a unique perspective and lens to approach my role and work as command surgeon at the preeminent National War College for the military. However, beyond all these experiences, it was a chance encounter with the National War College's most famous contemporary alumni that would change my career trajectory and make all the difference in my AI journey.

While volunteering to serve as the physician to provide medical support at the General Colin Powell dedication ceremony for the National War College's Library in Roosevelt Hall, I briefly met General Powell at the conclusion of the ceremony. Our interaction lasted only a few minutes, but during our chance encounter, I was the beneficiary of General Powell's magnanimous personality, attention, gracious spirit, generosity of time, and the benefit of his wise advice. After learning about my career, my role as command surgeon, and my pending matriculation to the Eisenhower School for National Security and Resource Strategy in 2017, General Powell convincingly suggested I instead attend his alma mater at the National Defense University, the National War College.

Suffice it to say, the serendipitous meeting with General Powell and his suggestion that I attend the National War College created a challenging dilemma for me since military medical officers did not customarily matriculate in the National War College. However, after having a discussion with the National Defense University dean of students and highlighting General Powell's suggestion—and because the Navy had not yet filled its allotted seats that year at the National War College—Dean John Yaeger made an exception. He granted me, the National Defense University command surgeon and naval medical officer, the opportunity to enter the National War College's class of 2018 as the only physician in a class of two hundred national security leaders.

The rest of the story was literally history. Building on my positive past experiences with graduate independent studies, leveraging a cadre of talented and well-connected National War College faculty, and taking advantage of the institution's unique history-based curriculum, I aimed to work on a thesis and research AI's role in military medicine.

AI and military medicine fit within the ethos of a national security strategy and were commensurate with the heritage of a graduate institution of national security policy that has had a significant impact on the world. Additionally, I advanced the idea that the nation's and its warfighters' health is a national security imperative. At every opportunity I shared how warfighter health, the military, and national security were inextricably connected and provided historical context to my colleagues, offering a unique medical history lens to our discussion and study of war.

Reducing Surgical Infections on the Battlefield: Dr. Joseph Lister

A watershed moment in the history of surgery, Dr. Joseph Lister introduced the idea of preventing surgical infections by bacteria in 1860. A young surgeon from the Edinburgh Royal Infirmary, Lister was influenced by Louis Pasteur's papers on bacteria.

Before Lister's work, surgeons rarely washed their hands, wore street clothes while operating, and freely circulated between the living patients they treated and the dead ones they dissected or autopsied. Before Lister, no surgeon risked opening an abdomen or entering a joint—on the battlefield or off. Surgical wound infections among soldiers spread from patient to patient like wildfire. Abscesses were left unopened and rarely drained, and most compound fractures resulted in eventual amputation. The death rate from major surgical operations or limb amputation hovered between 40 and 60 percent. Even simple procedures carried a high risk of death from infection.

By 1890, almost three decades after Lister introduced his theory, the whole world had accepted his theories, and medicine embarked on the era of antisepsis, revolutionizing the practice of surgery both in the military and among the civilian practice of medicine. Surgeons who embraced Lister's innovation and improved upon his discovery in antisepsis observed improved patient outcomes. This practice ushered in a new world of opportunity for patient care.

Revolutionary Vaccination and General George Washington

In 1776 smallpox devastated the Continental Army. Soon after the outbreak, General George Washington ordered the mandatory inoculation against smallpox for soldiers who had not gained prior immunity against the disease through infection. Through a procedure known during that era as variolation, individuals were intentionally exposed to a mild form of the smallpox virus. As a consequence of Washington's orders, the Continental Army was the first in the world to have an organized program to prevent smallpox.

Endemic diseases have always been a significant concern for the military, as well as potential exposures to lethal agents deliberately introduced into the environment through biological warfare or bioterrorism. In the age of synthetic biologics, genetically engineered novel threats are now possible. This threat has expanded the scope of military vaccine research and development.

The toll of history's worst epidemics, such as the Spanish flu, surpasses all the military deaths in World War I, World War II, the Korean conflict, and Vietnam combined. In fact, more person-days among US soldiers were lost to infection-borne disease than to bullets throughout the entire twentieth century.

Military research programs, driven primarily by the effects of infectious disease on military conflicts, have served an important role throughout history and have made significant contributions to medicine and, in particular, to vaccine development.

Throughout our seminar and small group discussions, I would politely point out to my fellow War College classmates how disease, germs, and illnesses often proved far more lethal to the warfighter than actual bullets. In fact, in 2018, my recounting of the Spanish flu's widespread and global devastation to my colleagues appeared to be received as fantasy. However, I remained adamant that pandemics represented a genuine national security threat. This observation was illustrated in vivid detail with the global COVID-19 pandemic.

Transforming Trauma Care: Blood Banks and Transfusion

During the American Civil War, we find two recorded cases of blood transfusion for treating bleeding following a leg amputation. By World War I, blood for transfusion was delivered to the front lines using citrate as a preservative and anticoagulant. The military carefully coordinated the distribution of blood and established specific indications for transfusion.

The United States Army was the first service to establish a military blood bank. Despite early challenges, the program became the starting point from which a much more massive initiative would develop to save countless lives on and off the battlefield.

The Iraq and Afghanistan wars challenged accepted concepts of trauma resuscitation and surgery. Only 10 percent of members of the United States Armed Forces wounded in Iraq and Afghanistan between 2003 and 2009 died compared with 24 percent in the first Gulf War (1990–1991) and the Vietnam War, in part because of novel utilization of blood transfusions and innovations in bleeding control.

The US military dedicated decades of work to shaping its current blood bank program into what it is today. The program continues to improve how blood is collected, stored, shipped, and transfused—and influences civilian practices. The military's continued modernization and standardization of its blood program still serve as a vanguard for best practices in critical medical therapy. In addition, military anesthesiologists pioneered an infrastructure that allows for the scaled medical and surgical capabilities that anesthesia facilitates.

SMARTER HEALTHCARE WITH AI

AI and Suicide Prevention

One of our focuses at the JAIC was suicide among our military service members. Suicide significantly leads the group of causes of death in the military at 28.1 percent. Data reveals that a member of the United States Armed Forces commits suicide every twenty-four hours, and a US veteran takes their own life every hour. This deeply rooted social crisis of suicide eludes solutions from experts and military leaders alike. Despite billions of dollars invested in suicide prevention programs, there seems to be limited impact or relief for active duty members of the Armed Forces and veterans.

Military medicine is at the forefront of addressing this crisis—one that is also experienced in the civilian world. The Centers for Disease Control and Prevention (CDC) reports[1] that suicide is one of the leading causes of all deaths in the United States. In 2021 nearly fifty thousand US residents died by suicide, approximately one death every eleven minutes. While people aged eighty-five and older have the highest suicide rates, youth suicide rates have increased over the past decade, with 23 percent of high school[2] students surveyed indicating they had seriously considered death by suicide in 2023.

Social media platforms, such as Facebook, employ an AI system programmed to spot potential suicidal language in users' posts. In some cases the system determines an individual is at risk and passes the information to a moderator, who may then alert authorities to intervene before a suicide or personal harm event occurs.

Facebook reported that in the fall of 2017, within a month, its AI system identified at-risk users through moderators and alerted first responders to intervene in one hundred cases of potential self-harm events that may have led to suicide.

In the military, Facebook's AI-assisted suicide alert system is one of many efforts to use AI to potentially help identify service members at risk for suicide as early as possible. In these instances researchers may use computers to sift massive amounts of data, such as EHRs, an individual's audio and video recordings, and social media posts to identify common attributes among people who attempted suicide. With this information algorithms can be developed to help predict which individuals are most likely to be at risk for suicide and deploy treatment and resources to help before another life is lost.

In recent years other AI-powered home-based virtual assistants such as Apple's Siri and Amazon's Alexa have directed users to the National Suicide Prevention Lifeline and have offered to connect users when they detect suicidal comments or questions emerging during engagement with the platform. The use of the word "suicide" or making statements that indicate individuals want to harm themselves triggers an intervention.

Top 5 Causes of Death in the United States Military	
Cause of Death	Percentage of US Military Deaths
1. Suicide	28.1%
2. Transport accidents	18.3%
3. Other accidents	9.3%
4. Combat	9%
5. Cancer	8%

Military medicine is entrusted with caring for the health of service members and family members. Defined as a population, the health outcomes of service members and their families are both the direct and indirect result of military medicine's collective effort of care. Therefore, military medicine aims to protect, preserve, and improve the health of service members and their families. This critical yet straightforward objective is consequential to every military unit's operational success and, by extension, a linchpin to our national security.

AI and the C.A.R.E. Model

If you can't measure something, you cannot improve it. This concept is central to almost every process in industry but eludes application in some aspects of civilian and military medicine. For this reason I adopted a particular strategy through my years of service and while serving in Africa during the Ebola epidemic: the C.A.R.E. model. This model has been tested for decades by cardiac surgeons and is regarded as the standard quality assessment tool in cardiac surgery.

The C.A.R.E. model's four-step process for quality improvement has a universal application. With vast datasets of healthcare information, AI can be used in medicine to augment health delivery using the C.A.R.E. model. The collection of data allows for machine learning. Analysis of collected data measured against established standards determined by evidence-based metrics could serve as the basis for personalized health on a scale never before realized. Adding a reporting and feedback process allows patients, individual providers, and groups to identify areas for improvement with higher fidelity than currently exists. For example, with AI's assistance, diet and behavior adjustments can be suggested before a patient slips from health into early illness.

In military applications, using available datasets and machine learning, patterns may be discovered with greater accuracy and scale. A service member's risk of injury or disease could be learned before deployment, possibly averting an expensive unplanned redeployment home and the consequent negative impact on a unit's mission success. The evaluation process allows further objective assessment and focuses on new quality improvement and health maintenance as prerequisites to readiness.

Inherent in the C.A.R.E. model is the ability to measure performance and the quality of health delivery and interventions. In the case of cardiac surgery, this process was partly responsible for an observed progressive drop in operative mortality from 1994 to 2003 in the United States, despite an increased predicted operative mortality during that period. The same quality improvements could be expected in service members' healthcare outcomes in military medicine.

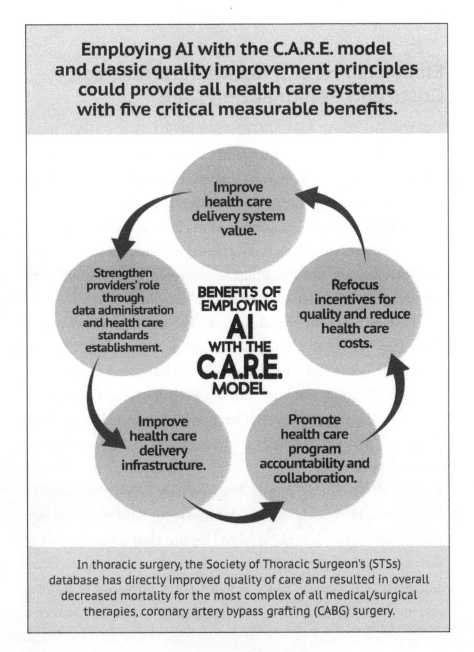

Employing AI with the C.A.R.E. model and classic quality improvement principles could provide all health care systems with five critical measurable benefits.

Improve health care delivery system value.

Strengthen providers' role through data administration and health care standards establishment.

BENEFITS OF EMPLOYING **AI** WITH THE **C.A.R.E.** MODEL

Refocus incentives for quality and reduce health care costs.

Improve health care delivery infrastructure.

Promote health care program accountability and collaboration.

In thoracic surgery, the Society of Thoracic Surgeon's (STSs) database has directly improved quality of care and resulted in overall decreased mortality for the most complex of all medical/surgical therapies, coronary artery bypass grafting (CABG) surgery.

The lessons learned in the quality improvement process and replication of the C.A.R.E. model with AI offer military and civilian healthcare systems the potential to achieve universal, value-based quality at lower cost and, consequently, to achieve the objectives of improved readiness and population health in military medicine.

Electronic Health Records: Reducing Costs and Personalizing Care

The Military Health System GENESIS EHR initiatives built upon previous legacy information systems to measurably enhance value, quality, and safety for the system's patients. As the EHR system is fully implemented throughout the military enterprise, AI technologies can specifically be leveraged. Employing AI will provide military medicine with improved healthcare delivery, reduced healthcare costs, increased accountability and collaboration, an improved healthcare delivery infrastructure, and more effective medical providers.

EHR is a big data breakthrough. The latest iterations of the technology have received praise and criticism. Indeed, the EHR has been cited in over 593 scholarly articles and attributed to improved physician efficiency and burnout. The EHR has also achieved one monumental accomplishment: it has provided an incredible amount of data to a patient's healthcare continuum. It is in the data that real value will be realized.

The EHR quickly moved from military to civilian medical applications. In fact, civilian healthcare systems have taken the ball and run with it. For example, at Johns Hopkins Hospital in Baltimore, Maryland, an AI-powered command center receives data from throughout the medical center to make a real impact on individual patients' lives. Since the hospital's investment in the AI-enhanced command center in 2016, there has been a 60 percent increase in the hospital's ability to accept and care for complex cancer patients. Johns Hopkins also observed a 25 percent reduction in emergency room boarding time and the transition time a patient spends in the ER after admission before being transferred to an inpatient unit within the hospital. The hospital also achieved a 60 percent reduction in operating room hold times. Overall, the investment in AI-leveraged technology has already improved the efficiency and workflow at Johns Hopkins Hospital, and improvements continue to be realized.

In 2012 a rural hospital in southwest Michigan invested in EHR and enhanced the system with AI technology in 2016. By enabling automated data entry and analysis of routine patient monitoring, nurses could spend more time on patient care. Additionally, an AI-driven early-warning system built into the patient monitoring system reduced the hospital's code blues—the clinical term ascribed for cardiac or respiratory arrest patients—by 56 percent. The system accurately identified subtle changes in a patient's vital signs and assigned risk scores to patients. This information helped nurses prioritize patient care, reduce complications, and avert code blues among the patient population.

The AI Medical Revolution Is Already Here

[If] you're arguing against AI, then you're arguing against safer cars that aren't going to have accidents, and you're arguing against being able to better diagnose people when they're sick.
—MARK ZUCKERBERG

Will AI replace physicians? Perhaps. The day may come soon when patients feel more comfortable receiving care and information about their health from a computer than from another human being. No one could predict that we would no longer need the library card catalog to find information in a library or rely on a platform called Google or ChatGPT to obtain information about many everyday issues. Yet that day has come.

Experts predict rapid progress will continue accelerating AI advances in the coming years. AI could be a transformative technology in medicine on par with, and perhaps superseding, anesthesia, vaccines, antisepsis, and blood transfusion. AI technologies include cognitive, RPA, autonomics, machine learning, and deep learning. Future-oriented strategies are being implemented to leverage AI to create a better, stronger, and more relevant military medical force to support the health, readiness, and resilience of the warfighter and their families.

To date, significant technical progress in AI has been driven by data science, algorithms, and advanced computer hardware. Potential applications in healthcare now make this era dramatically different. A confluence of three powerful forces engenders society to embrace new health-centric approaches enabled by advances in AI. These powerful forces include frustration with current legacy medical systems, the ubiquity of networked smart devices in society, and the acclimation and widespread use of at-home AI-enhanced convenience services like those currently provided through commercial industries.

The application of AI technologies in military medicine is already improving individual service members' health and readiness, as well as the health of the service population.

Go!

The board game Go has exponentially more mathematical and strategic depth than chess—I have enjoyed playing Go with my daughter a few times. In 2014 a computer beat a human Go champion ten years earlier than had been predicted by the programmer who designed the world's best Go-playing program. This kind of intelligent human-behavior simulation in computers defines AI.

Computers that beat real humans at Go, self-driving cars, advanced facial recognition, and almost all other AI advances are based on decades-old breakthroughs that leading computer scientists pioneered. Computers are less sophisticated than the human brain. Consequently, teaching computers to learn "like a human" is comparatively more difficult. General AI, or human-level artificial general intelligence, is the ability of computers to learn and behave with the natural fluidity of the human brain. Complete knowledge of how the actual human brain works is still limited. Therefore, experts consider simulating computer behavior to learn and function like the human mind to be decades away.

Narrow AI, however, focuses on teaching computers limited sequential tasks. This kind of present-day machine learning contributes much to the contemporary advances realized in AI, such as self-driving cars. The current lexicon of AI innovation is based on deep learning, a type of machine learning that has existed for decades. Progress in deep learning will lead to many future breakthroughs in narrow AI in the coming years as previous barriers come down.

Now many of computer science's early limitations in computing power, data sources, and expertise have been mitigated. The difference today is the convergence of factors that make the potential for AI more advanced than it was in the past.

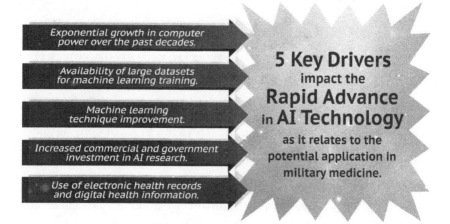

The value at stake from AI technologies varies widely between different industries. However, based on its market size, pain points, and willingness to invest in AI technologies and realize a return on investments to improve value, health care, in particular, is primed to follow the wave of AI adoption.

When health is absent, wisdom cannot reveal itself, art cannot become manifest, strength cannot fight, wealth becomes useless, and intelligence cannot be applied.

—HEROPHILUS OF CHALCEDON, GREEK PHYSICIAN AND ANATOMIST

Literally interpreted, Herophilus says that health transcends education, culture, and economics. In the military, the stakes for health are even higher. The health and fitness of the warfighter are essential for mission success, national security, and the preservation of our national interests.

The DoD directs and finances military healthcare through its agencies and has, over the years, implemented various health information system initiatives with new visions, goals, and objectives, including creating fully integrated digital hospitals and care platforms to care for warfighters and their families in the modern era.

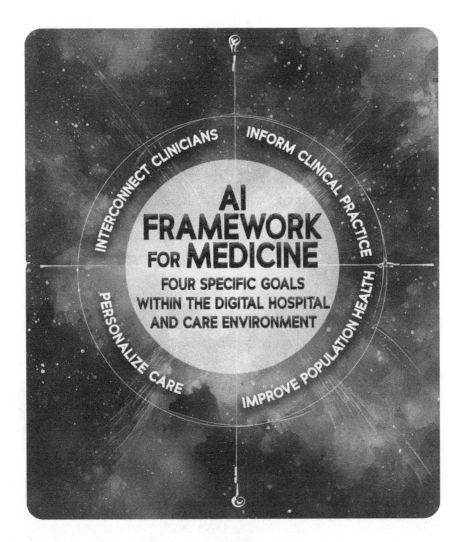

Designing Ways to Health

The DHA's primary objective is to maintain the health of military personnel so they can execute their military missions efficiently and deliver healthcare during wartime. Operating around the world, the DHA currently serves nearly 10 million beneficiaries through 56 hospitals, 365 clinics, and contracted care purchased from private civilian providers. The DHA employs more than 58,369 civilians and 86,007 military personnel.

Five crucial steps have been offered in designing ways to succeed in the strategic application of AI in military medicine to achieve improved health, service readiness, and population health. Based on cutting-edge research in the field of machine- and human-interactions, these steps have been dubbed the "Fourth Industrial Revolution" and defined at the 2016 World Economic Forum Meeting in Davos, Switzerland, as "the wave of technological advances that are changing the way we live, work, stay alive, and interact with each other and machines."

The Limits of Artificial Intelligence

We tend to overestimate the effect of a technology in the short run and underestimate the effect in the long run.

—ROY AMARA

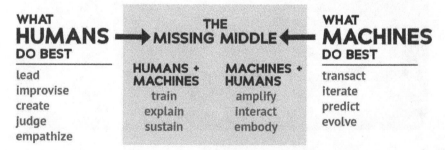

The missing middle — the tasks best done through man-machine collaboration

Daugherty, Paul R. and Wilson, H. James. Human + Machine: Reimagining Work in the Age of AI *(United States: Harvard Business Review Press, 2018).*

Despite sensational claims to the contrary, it is unlikely that machines will take over the world and forever displace humans in the workplace. In the case of AI, systems are enhancing the skills of humans rather than replacing them, leading to more productive work. The human brain is very complicated and still needs to be fully understood. There are, therefore, essential activities that will remain uniquely human. These include leading, empathizing, creating, and exercising judgment. Machine and artificial learning systems have also been proven to perform certain activities more efficiently. These activities include transactions (e.g., ATMs), iteration (e.g., financial investments), and prediction (e.g., weather forecasts).

In between these two spectrums of activities exists a middle category best described as hybrid activities in which humans may complement machines and machines enhance and augment human capabilities. In this so-called "missing middle" category, humans and machines could best be described as symbiotic partners, each allowing the other to achieve higher performance and achievement. The tasks and activities performed within the missing middle include training, explaining, amplifying, interacting, embodying, and sustaining. These areas have the most significant potential for AI application in designing ways to promote health.

Consider this example. A person wakes up one morning feeling ill. He explains to his AI-enhanced home platform that he is not feeling well. A series of sensors in his home interact with him to determine that, indeed, he has a fever, an elevated heart rate, and a slightly elevated respiratory rate. His AI-enhanced platform is trained to recognize his voice and detects that his voice is slightly distorted. His AI-enhanced platform makes a telehealth connection, and a virtual visit is established with a nurse practitioner who confirms his symptoms. Additional diagnostic tests during the encounter, including a rapid strep test processed through the AI-enhanced platform, amplify the nurse practitioner's assessment, and the results return positive for streptococcus infection.

Through the established AI-enhanced connection, the nurse practitioner explains to the patient the diagnosis of strep throat. Based on his known drug allergies and established medical history, she advises him that appropriate antibiotic treatment will be delivered via express courier service to his home within hours. She informs him that a follow-up visit will be performed within twenty-four hours.

The nurse practitioner has embodied all the elements of a professional, compassionate, comprehensive care plan and will have the opportunity to rapidly assess the effectiveness of the treatment delivered within hours of the encounter because the AI-enhanced platform will continue to collect and record real-time vital sign data on the patient and report changes to the provider. Additionally, the patient will have the opportunity during the follow-up encounters to subjectively report if he feels better or needs additional assistance, requiring a visit to his primary care provider or the emergency room.

Indeed, interest in AI is at its apogee in most industries now. Companies in many sectors have advanced AI-focused initiatives. What is needed is the management of expectations, patience, and dedication to strategic experimentation.

Studies reveal that the inherent potential of AI to transform industries, particularly healthcare, is significant indeed. McKinsey Global Institute found 45 percent of work activities could potentially be automated, and of those activities, machine learning could enable 80 percent. The report highlights that healthcare has captured less than 30 percent of the potential from its data and analytics investments. Barriers such as demonstration of clinical utility, interoperability, and data sharing remain challenges.

Research suggests that adopting a portfolio approach to AI projects with a diverse cadre of plans may generate both quick wins and long-term projects focused on transforming end-to-end workflow.

For quick wins in military medicine, the use of recent advances in speech, vision, and language understanding is critical. For example, an AI-enhanced voice interface could help pharmacists look up substitute medications; provide tools to assist administrators with scheduling internal meetings, clinic appointments, and operating room workflow efficiency; and, overall, save resources in time and human capital.

AI quick-win initiatives in military medicine will not be universally transformational. However, they will help engender consensus and interest in the potential of AI. More importantly, smaller AI projects will help the organization gain invaluable experience with large-scale data gathering, labeling, processing, and harnessing the skills that the military medicine enterprise must master before embarking on more ambitious transformational AI projects.

In military medicine, long-term projects will go beyond point optimization to fundamentally rethinking end-to-end processes. However, the most significant impact and value realized through AI will be in new care-delivery processes. For example, aspects of a business process, such as claims processing for veterans, may be automated entirely using speech and vision understanding to expedite the process. This will save time and costs while significantly improving service members' satisfaction.

Personalized treatment plans could be designed ubiquitously throughout the military medicine enterprise by machine learning tools. This would enhance therapy efficiency by tailoring treatment to specific patients' needs and medical conditions. Additionally, AI-enhanced insights could be gained on the battlefield from sensors applied to the warfighter to help triage care more effectively in the field and prepare providers for definitive care of the injured, ill, or traumatized patients throughout the continuum of their recovery.

AI-enhanced population-health analyses could allow TRICARE, the government's managed health insurance program, to reduce hospitalization and treatment costs by encouraging care providers to manage patients' wellness more effectively. Companies such as Google have already learned that building such high-value workflow automation requires deep organizational skills in training machine learning algorithms and technology.

Indeed, AI has transformed healthcare and will continue to do so. However, for the Military Health System to harness AI's transformative powers, its application must begin with a strategy that realizes its limits, invests in areas where it will make the most impact, and embraces a portfolio approach rather than one big win.

The Future Is Now

The saddest aspect of life right now is that science gathers knowledge faster than society gathers wisdom.

—ISAAC ASIMOV

5
KEY
AI ADVANCEMENT
ISSUES OF EQUAL IMPORTANCE.

As the AI transformation of health care calls for the application of new technologies, both military and civilian medical systems must move forward with prudence.

PRIVACY: We must establish guidelines, rules, and regulations to cover the risks associated with AI as data is collected, stored, transferred, and manipulated and add additional layers of protection for the handling of confidential health information.

ACCURACY: AI technologies are dependent on data for accurate machine learning. Potential implications for system biases or errors to occur must be mitigated with measures that ensure good, safe, and reliable data governance.

SAFETY: As AI technologies advance, security must be guaranteed so that harm to patients is minimized, especially in the case of AI-enhanced platforms that are used in the care of patients with suicide risk.

RESPONSIBILITY: Because AI assessments may differ from clinical opinions, it will be necessary to have clear guidelines for how to proceed to keep the safety and care of the patient at the forefront.

KNOWLEDGE GAP: Much is still unknown about how AI technologies evolve and what the future will bring. There will always be a risk that the technology becomes uncontrollable. It is paramount that we continue to invest in research and development to better understand and manage AI technologies and to be leaders in innovation of the application of the technology in military and civilian medicine.

Future applications of AI technologies are likely to be more robust as natural market forces drive its advancement in other industries such as finance, energy, and retail. And AI will have significant implications for both military and civilian medicine. Coupled with the unique abundance of data stored on service members, AI may help understand disease at its fundamental level to facilitate better treatment and therapeutics to help patients more efficiently.

The private sector has been leveraging AI in healthcare to establish quicker diagnoses, better treatment plans, and improved health insurance. The application of machine learning to the radiological interpretation of CT scans has had a significant impact on surgery as applying algorithms to radiologic imaging can detect cancer earlier than humans can.

Physicians are using AI to tailor treatment plans for individual patients and improve operations. They are also identifying public health threats and at-risk patients earlier than before. This is helping improve population health more efficiently and on a larger scale than ever before.

As a tool to augment care, AI has the potential to consolidate biological data, physician data, subjective patient data inputs, treatment, and diagnoses. A use case at Walter Reed Medical Center demonstrates how the Department of Veterans Affairs is currently partnering with the DoD to use AI technologies to better predict medical complications and improve treatment of severe combat wounds, ideally leading to improved patient outcomes, faster healing, and lower costs.

Ultimately, applying AI in military medicine will improve service readiness, service member population health, and DoD time, money, and resource savings. Without a doubt, this will fuel a healthcare revolution in civilian medicine as well.

AI is fundamentally transforming the relationship among patients, providers, and machines. This trend will only continue in the coming years and will be more pronounced among younger generations, particularly the millennial generation, which now fills most of the ranks in the services. For this reason innovators in both military and civilian healthcare systems must become adept at designing, training, and collaborating with AI systems to achieve enhanced performance across the spectrum of healthcare delivery.

NOTES

Stiglitz, J. E., "The $3 Trillion War" (2008), https://doi.org/10.7916/
D8HX1PHC.

"Joseph Lister and the Story of Antiseptic Surgery," *Hektoen International* 6, no. 3 (Summer 2014), https://hekint.org/2017/01/22/
joseph-lister-and-the-story-of-antiseptic-surgery/.

"U.S. Military and Vaccine History," History of Vaccines, https://
cpp-hov.netlify.app/vaccines-101/how-are-vaccines-made/
us-military-and-vaccine-history/.

"Damage Control Resuscitation for Patients with Major Trauma," *BMJ* (June 2009), https://www.bmj.com/content/338/bmj.b1778.long.

Söderlund, M., & Oikarinen, E. L., "Service Encounters with Virtual Agents: An Examination of Perceived Humanness as a Source of Customer Satisfaction, *European Journal of Marketing* 55, no. 13, 94–121.

Shead, Sam, "Elon Musk Says Mark Zuckerberg's Understanding of AI Is 'Limited' after the Facebook CEO Called His Warnings 'Irresponsible,'" Entrepreneur, https://www.entrepreneur.com/business-news/
elon-musk-says-mark-zuckerbergs-understanding-of-ai-is/297729.

Tetteh, Hassan, "AI in Defense," JAIC, https://www.ai.mil/blog_02_26_20-
jaic_warfighter_health.html.

"Instabase Named to Guidewire Insurtech Vanguards Program," Business Wire, https://www.businesswire.com/news/home/20220615005429/en/Instabase-Named-to-Guidewire-Insurtech-Vanguards-Program.

"INBT Seminar: Captain (Dr.) Hassan A. Tetteh," Johns Hopkins Institute for NanoBioTechnology, https://inbt.jhu.edu/event/inbt-seminar-capt-dr-hassan-a-tetteh/?instance_id=52.

Tetteh, Hassan, "AI in Defense," JAIC, https://www.ai.mil/blog_02_26_20-jaic_warfighter_health.html.

Grant, P. J., "Third Party Collections" (2008), https://doi.org/10.21236/ada483179.

"Contact," World Leaders Forum Dubai, https://worldleadersforumdubai.com/contact/.

Abdallah, C., "Wednesday Communiqué, 2/29/2012," 2012.

Leary, P. A., "Selecting Continuing Education," *Journal of the American Dental Association* (2017), https://doi.org/10.1016/j.adaj.2017.05.016.

Tetteh, Hassan, "AI in Defense," JAIC, https://www.ai.mil/blog_02_26_20-jaic_warfighter_health.html.

AN AI LIFEBOAT: MEDICAL IMAGING CLASSIFICATION

When I was first introduced to the DoD and the JAIC, they were not really looking at the supporting roles of AI technology in medicine, but more at how to make autonomous weapons, radar, cyber enhancements, and those kinds of applications. However, the organization knew inherently that medicine was important and wanted to make a case for funding AI initiatives in the health space that would directly impact the warfighter. They saw that AI could transform the EHR, but from a warfighting standpoint, they asked, what was the advantage?

My experience as a ship's surgeon answered their question. During the nearly two years I spent on an aircraft carrier, I spent nineteen months at sea. The problem with our deployment was that we were always out to sea. Our return to shore wasn't predictable. Often, young service members came to me with lumps and bumps, little moles, and concerns of that nature. There were a couple of ways to handle these matters. I could say, "Well, we'll just wait until we get to port, and then we'll do a biopsy."

However, I was a young surgeon interested in really helping people. I was concerned because I knew that young people could get cancers. The reality is that most people on aircraft carriers, especially if they're working on the flight deck, have quite a bit of exposure to the sun. They're out there—fully exposed, no trees or shade. The only things to give them any cover are the clouds—and technically, clouds don't protect people from the UV rays that cause cancers.

So young people came to me with unusual-looking moles and blemishes on their skin. I decided to biopsy them, resect them, fix the samples in a preservative formula, and then send them off the ship to a pathologist. You can imagine the logistics of that. Depending on where we were, that biopsy could fly around the world before getting to a pathologist. By the time it was read and transmitted back to us with a benign or malignant result, a lot of time had passed. In some cases we would wait months.

There was one case I'll never forget. A young man, a pilot in his late twenties, had a lesion on his inner thigh. It was very prominent and firm—a little unusual. It didn't look like the typical benign lesion. When I removed it, I told him about my concerns. When I got the results back, he had already left the ship. The results showed it was a malignant histiocytoma, a very aggressive type of malignancy that can spread. This young pilot needed treatment right away.

It took a lot of effort to hunt him down. When I did, I explained what I'd learned and told him that he needed treatment. Ultimately, he found his way into the hands of an oncologist and received proper care. But here was a young man who might not have received treatment if, one, I hadn't been doing the biopsies; two, I hadn't resected his biopsy; three, I hadn't sent it off the ship and received the results; and four, I hadn't made the very conscientious attempt to follow up on the results.

Results weren't always forthcoming. In this case I had to play Sherlock Holmes to find them, but not finding them could have been lethal for this young man.

ARMing Military Medicine

I shared this story with the people in the JAIC when they asked about the connection among AI, warfighter readiness, and medical care. I told them how an existing AI solution would have made a difference in this young sailor's case: the augmented reality microscope (ARM).

Google prototyped this microscope with the DoD. Using AI enhancements, the microscope facilitates classifying and identifying tissue samples—a boon to cancer diagnoses. These microscopes were specifically configured to detect breast cancer, prostate cancer, lymphoma, and colon cancer. When slides are put underneath this microscope, it draws circles around abnormal cells and alerts the pathologist to the abnormalities. It is faster, more accurate, and allows pathologists to handle more throughput. As part of the team conducting an independent assessment of the ARM, I saw a couple of cases where the pathologist had missed an abnormality, but the ARM detected it—and the patients received the care they needed. In 2022 we published a paper highlighting our findings in the *Journal of Pathology Informatics*.[3] It explained how these microscopes were more accurate than pathology specialists at detecting particular cancers. I remember telling my colleagues at the JAIC,

> Can you imagine if we'd had this microscope on that aircraft
> carrier when I cared for the pilot with the lesion on his thigh?
> And if we'd had the lab techs who could fix the tissue from the

biopsy and do the staining and preparation? We could have put it under this microscope and looked at it right there. If we'd had this interface on that ship, we could have seen that there was an abnormality and made an early diagnosis rather than waiting and worrying for weeks and months. We could have protected sailors and pilots and found them the care they needed before it was too late. By the time he was treated, this young pilot could very well have been at a point where his cancer was too far advanced. The Navy could have lost a great asset in a pilot—and a young man, whose life might have been saved, could have been lost instead.

That was when the folks at the JAIC started to understand. They saw the direct application of AI to warfighter health and service readiness.

CNBC covered the Google/DoD ARM collaboration and the paper we released in September 2023. I found this excerpt from the CNBC article especially interesting. It's also interesting that the physician in this article, Niels Olson, was named "Sailor of the Year" for the entire Navy in 2021.[4]

Few understand the challenges pathologists face quite like Dr. Niels Olson, the chief medical officer of the Defense Innovation Unit, or DIU, at the DoD. The DIU was created in 2015 as a way for the military to integrate cutting-edge technology developed by the commercial world. The organization negotiates contracts with companies so they can collaborate and circumvent long bureaucratic hang-ups.

Olson is a pathologist. Before beginning his role at the DIU, he served in the US Navy. In 2018 he was sent to Guam, a US island territory in Micronesia, where he worked as the laboratory medical director and blood bank director in the Naval Hospital.

During his two years in Guam, Olson was one of two pathologists on the island and the only pathologist in the Naval Hospital. This meant he was often making major decisions and diagnoses on his own.

"It's not just your job to say, 'This is cancer, it's this kind of cancer.' Part of the job is saying, 'It's absolutely not cancer,' and that can be nerve-wracking when you're alone," Olson told CNBC in an interview. "I would have loved to have an augmented reality microscope in Guam, just so there'd be somebody, something else helping."

The ARM is meant to serve as a second line of defense for pathologists, and Olson said it would not replace the doctors themselves. He added that the obvious initial use case for the microscope would be in smaller, remote labs, and it could also serve as a resource for pathology residents in training.

But Olson had dreamed up a tool like the ARM long before his time in Guam. On August 10, 2016, while working as a resident at the Naval Medical Center in San Diego, Olson decided to message a connection he had at Google. In the email, which CNBC viewed, Olson described a rough idea of what a microscope like the ARM could be.

For a while Olson said he heard nothing. But months later he was standing in a Google office building in Mountain View, California, crammed in a locked room to which only a few people at the company had access. There, he watched as an early AI-powered microscope successfully identified cancer on a small set of slides he had brought.

Olson said the room was sweltering because everyone inside was "pumped."

"I don't want to say it's quite like seeing your kid for the first time, but it was sort of like, this is awesome, this is going to be a thing," Olson said.

Around the time he was sent to Guam, a product manager at the DIU came across Olson's research. The pair wrote an article together in 2019 about how the DoD and Silicon Valley could collaborate to leverage AI. They said the federal government has millions of patients enrolled in its healthcare systems, which means it boasts "the most comprehensive healthcare dataset in the world." That data has obvious commercial use.

"Big data is what Silicon Valley does best, and the potential for spillover into civilian healthcare systems is vast," they wrote.

Shortly after that, the DIU began looking for commercial partners to help build and test the ARM. The organization picked the optical technology company Jenoptik to handle the hardware, and after evaluating thirty-nine companies, it selected Google to develop the software.

Aashima Gupta, global director of healthcare strategy and solutions at Google Cloud, said the company has since launched four algorithms for the ARM, which can identify breast cancer, cervical cancer, prostate cancer, and mitosis. The AI models are trained on data from the DIU, and Gupta said Google employees and Google infrastructure need access to it.

"It's encrypted all the way," Gupta told CNBC in an interview. "From how the data is collected to how it is stored and analyzed—and anything in between."

There's a huge amount of testing to be done.

With the hardware and the software in order, the DIU has been conducting initial research to test the ARM's efficacy.

In the fall of 2022, the organization published a peer-reviewed paper in the *Journal of Pathology Informatics*. The paper found that the breast cancer AI algorithm performed reasonably well across many samples. Still, there are caveats, said David Jin, the lead author of the paper and the deputy director for AI assessment at the DoD's Chief Digital and Artificial Intelligence Office.

The paper specifically examined how well the AI performed when detecting breast cancer metastasis in lymph nodes, and Jin said it did better on certain types of cells than others. He said the study is promising, but there's still a vast amount of rigorous testing to be done before it can support pathologists with real patient care.

"Something like this has an extreme potential for benefit, but also there's a lot of risks," as it would change how cancer diagnosis is done, Jin told CNBC in an interview.

Olson, who returned from Guam and began working at the DIU in 2020, is also listed as an author of the paper. He said independent assessments of the other three models, for prostate cancer, mitosis, and cervical cancer, have not been carried out at the DIU yet.

Research with the ARM is ongoing, and the DIU is also soliciting feedback from organizations such as Mitre and health systems such as Veterans Affairs. There is work to be done, but since the DIU has validated the initial concept, the organization is beginning to consider scaling the technology and collaborating with regulators.

The DIU negotiated agreements with Google and Jenoptik that will allow the technology to be distributed military-wide and commercially. The DIU hopes to make the ARM available to all government users through the General Services Administration website.

Nadeem Zafar of VA Puget Sound said that the ARM will ultimately aid pathologists, but the general public will benefit most from the technology. He said the ARM's accuracy, speed, and cost-effectiveness will all contribute to better care.

"AI is here, and it's going to keep developing," Zafar said. "The point is not to be afraid of these technologies, but to triage them to the best use for our medical and healthcare needs."

Project DARWIN: AI and the Evolution of Cancer Diagnosis

Another initiative my colleagues at the JAIC and I came up with was Project DARWIN: Digital AI-AcceleRation With Imaging IntegratioN. Formerly known as the Armed Forces Research Institute, the Joint Pathology Center (JPC) has a warehouse full of pathology slides of unique and rare tumors. Pathology slides have been sent to the JPC for over a century. They are all cataloged. When we couldn't figure out the pathology of something when I was a medical student at SUNY Downstate Health Sciences University in Brooklyn or when I was in my medical fellowship in Minnesota, we would send a sample to the JPC. Usually, we would get results back identifying what it most likely was. The JPC has a database of the rarest pathologies on the planet.

We embarked on one such project with Google and Jenoptik. It entailed digitizing one small set of slides by photographing the glass slides and converting them to an electronic format. Using AI, a physician in any location could upload a digital photograph of a pathology, match it to this digitized database of slides, and rapidly determine certain cancers. This resolution would have otherwise taken weeks or months.

I pushed hard to get Project DARWIN up and running. Political forces being what they were, this project was not implemented during my tenure at the JAIC. But I still have hope. People in pathology, radiology, and oncology know that the collection of pathology slides at the JPC is an invaluable resource. It's an enormous repository of untapped potential. Though very well known, many medical professionals feel that it's not being utilized to its full potential. Investing in digitizing a good portion of these slides and creating more models to interface with the ARM and future technologies could have revolutionary effects on healthcare delivery.

PROJECT DARWIN

Because the use of clinically validated AI will be a driver for great outcomes by reducing human error, early exposure to AI will ensure a medical force is ready for the future of medicine. Using clinically validated AI to improve the healthcare experience will increase patient satisfaction and clinician workflow by automating routine functions, freeing them from mundane tasks, and providing daily evidence that they are working in a cutting-edge organization.

On August 3, 2020—six days before the World Health Organization (WHO) declared COVID-19 a pandemic—the Defense Innovation Board made a series of recommendations to enhance the JPC, the world's largest tissue archive. Within a month, $20 million had been secured for a pilot digitization effort, and the DHA was tasked to oversee the pilot, led by the JPC, with the Defense Digital Service assisting. This project could still pave the way for the large-scale digitization of the JPC's holdings, enabling the production of datasets to train machine learning algorithms to classify many of the diseases diagnosed by histomorphology—most importantly, most, if not all, forms of cancer.

The holdings include an Enterprise Clinical Imaging Archive with seven hundred million radiology studies. In addition, the Military Health System Information Platform data warehouse holds copies of every DHA record, which could be integrated.

In collaboration with the JAIC, the JPC could have digitized a de-identified version of data elements in the pathology reports for cases. The digitized holdings could be made available to other government biomedical research and development efforts and serve as a resource for training algorithms.

For decades, the JPC received cases from around the world. By digitizing the slides from these cases, the Military Health System could harness the potential of this rich data for the benefit of our service members, their families, and society.

As I mentioned, during the pandemic, this repository had COVID-19 samples collected decades ago. Had these been available electronically via an AI-enhanced network, the development of the COVID-19 vaccine might have taken even less time than it did.

Educational institutions and commercial entities are already working to digitize pathology slides sourced elsewhere on a smaller scale. In February 2023 Yale School of Medicine reported that Yale New Haven Health had digitized close to sixty thousand histology glass slides from its own system and from outside institutions. Ohio State University Comprehensive Cancer Center and the University of Iowa Healthcare Carver School of Medicine Division of Anatomic Pathology provide scanning services to create digital whole-slide images from glass slides.[5]

Commercial organizations developing AI technology for digitizing pathology slides include Intel and Wistrom, which recently released a white paper that concluded, "Digital pathology has the potential to deliver incredible innovations in AI-enabled diagnoses for healthcare and research organizations all over the globe. In the future, hospitals worldwide may be able to use this technology to bring more detailed and accurate analysis to doctors and researchers. The goal is to enable AI technologies to give more patients better access to diagnosis and treatment, which is essential to address an increase in global cancer rates and a shortage of pathologists worldwide."

When I was with the JAIC, politics and competing interests came into play when we proposed Project DARWIN. There was a lot of protectionism around this vast repository of pathology slides, which did not make much sense to me. Some brought up the issue of patient privacy. However, we had found a process to de-identify personal information from slides offered for digitization. We can even use AI to anonymize the data. Even if we know that this is Jane Smith's tumor, that's inconsequential and irrelevant. But if you have a bunch of Jane Smiths with this precise cancer, you can train the models and develop the interface to help with cancer detection and inform treatment and therapy.

We recruited a cadre of people who agreed with the plan. We sent a proposal to the White House to see if we could get funding. We had some interest, but regrettably, the plan never launched because, for whatever reason, too many custodians of the slides were protecting this data. I'll call them antibodies to progress.

My team and I had a friend in the White House who was interested in helping us with Project DARWIN. I talked to him while I was working on this chapter of the book. He said, "To this day, I'm scratching my head—I just don't understand why we didn't make progress with this."

Ahead of the Curve

Another project I had hoped to get off the ground while at the JAIC would have used AI to help predict and treat lung cancer in our service members and veterans. In many ways, we at the JAIC were ahead of the AI curve in medicine. In 2018 some of my colleagues at Johns Hopkins and I submitted a grant proposal to the DoD to fund our project to develop algorithms to enhance the analysis of CT scans for the chest.

We had a cohort of patients with a cancer—chest cancer, thoracic cancer, or lung cancer. After these patients received chemotherapy or surgery, we scanned them every six months or so to see if there was a recurrence. This is a typical procedure. Once a patient has surgery or chemotherapy, we wait a few months and do another imaging study to see if any recurring cancer can be detected.

Within our patient cohort, we found both patients with a recurrence and others without. We also had a computer scan the images using AI algorithms to detect cancer recurrence. We adjusted for many of the common variables and challenges that occur when looking at disparate images taken on different machines using different techniques. In our pilot study with our limited sample size, we found that the computer platform, the AI, could detect cancer recurrence as much as eighteen months before a radiologist could. Why? Because the AI detected abnormalities in the imaging on a pixel level. This demonstrated great potential with AI technology, and in 2018 our AI was less robust than it is now.

We had compelling, statistically significant evidence. So we submitted our grant. We were confident we would get the funding, but we did not. The DoD gave us good and helpful feedback and stated our studies were very compelling. However, they wanted to see more data, which was ironic because we were requesting more funding to enroll more patients and get more data. Well, this was pre-pandemic and pre-ChatGPT. Clearly now, a study like this would have much more interest and be more appropriate for funding.

Indeed, the private sector has already realized the potential of using AI to enhance imaging and diagnoses. They are already developing MRI machines incorporating nascent AI into the hardware and software of diagnostic tools for screening and evaluating patients.

This AI technology has already been developed and is in use. If the DoD were to harness this vast resource, it could not only save lives but also cut costs. It would be a valuable tool in preserving warfighter health and readiness. It would also ensure the civilians it protects have access to faster and more accurate diagnoses and treatment. It will only take a little bit of an investment to get it up and running.

Incorporating AI into healthcare delivery is one way to address the need for more healthcare workers. The WHO predicts we will be short fifteen million healthcare professionals by 2030. For me, however, it all comes back to that young man, that young pilot, and all the other sailors I cared for on that aircraft carrier. I'm thinking about how we can save lives, translate that onto the battlefield, and share it with civilian medicine like the other developments in military medicine that have led the way in advancing medical breakthroughs.

NOTE

"AI-Powered Microscope Helps Doctors Spot Cancer," DiversityMD, https://diversitymd.com/blog/ai-powered-microscope-helps-doctors-spot-cancer/.

CHAPTER 4

HEALTH RECORDS
ANALYSIS

I t was ironic. I'm a fully informed informaticist and an AI practitioner. I had a leadership role in the Warfighter Health Mission at the JAIC. I consider myself reasonably healthy, yet I was steeped in frustration. Here I was, recently retired after a twenty-five-year career in the Navy and looking to set up my healthcare with the VA. Not only was I unable to navigate the VA's system with ease, but I also ran into roadblocks—from filing documents and documenting my disabilities and health conditions to scheduling appointments and going through the adjudication process. All of this showed me that there's ample room for improvement. After making several phone calls and not making any progress, I walked into the Washington, DC, VA facility, hoping to talk to someone and get some assistance. I was informed that nobody could help me and that I had to set up an appointment online. The earliest available face-to-face appointment was many months away—and the earliest virtual appointment was several weeks away. I made both of those appointments. That was when I fully understood and appreciated the pain points veterans talk about.

In my frustration I called more and more numbers. I finally contacted someone, Christopher, who was extremely helpful. He worked at the Roanoke, Virginia, VA facility. It so happened that the next day, I was planning to visit my son Edmund, who was in his freshman year of college in North Carolina. I asked Christopher, "Would it be all right if I stopped by your office tomorrow to visit?" He said, "Absolutely! We're open."

It was refreshing and comforting that he could do that for me. So I made a pit stop in Roanoke on my drive to North Carolina. I went to the VA facility. Everyone there was pleasant and very helpful. It was a bit of a journey, but when we met, Christopher shared which documents I needed to complete and how to complete some of them online and told me how he could help.

It dawned on me that there are clearly geographical differences in the services, patient care, and human connections one can find. I was very fortunate that I could drive down to Roanoke. But the whole experience reinforced the fact that there is a lot of room in the system for improvement—and AI has a significant role.

AI certainly is not a panacea or a silver bullet. However, the work that we were doing with health records at the JAIC, though somewhat abstract, could make lives easier, care more accessible, and costs lower for the VA.

While I was working on health records analysis at the JAIC, I began to understand the challenges that our service members have when engaging with the military's health systems, especially when they have sustained some sort of injury that makes them unable to do their jobs or, like me, when they retired and made the transition to the VA for healthcare. When I retired in 2023 and began to make that transition personally, I had the opportunity to fully understand the frustrations of transitioning to the VA for services.

Those injured and awaiting adjudication of what will happen to the rest of their careers are subjected to numerous tests and evaluations before a determination is rendered. This state of limbo is frustrating for the patient, their family, their peers, and their commanding officers. That's why we adopted the MERIT initiative, the Medical Evaluation Readiness Information Toolset.

MERIT: Medical Evaluation Readiness Information Toolset

In today's healthcare world, imagining life without electronic health records (EHRs), telehealth, and remote monitoring tools is impossible. These have increased patient care, quality, access, and efficiency. What if we could scan a complete medical record and provide treatment recommendations that would change the course of a disease and prolong a service member's career with medical evaluation readiness information tools?

During our tenure at the JAIC, my JAIC colleague Michelle Padgett and I collaborated on the Medical Evaluation Readiness Information Toolset (MERIT). This AI-enhanced approach to the EHR aims to improve service members' readiness by leveraging AI and health data analytics to empower early intervention for those at risk of entering the military's complicated disability system.

We evolved from standalone use to complex perspectives with summary and individual real-time data that provides a common operating picture for the patient, provider commander, and senior leaders. We know the health of service members is vital to force readiness. MERIT is establishing a predictive model to analyze data to provide indicators of a service member's health status, which is critical to our national security initiatives.

When service members cannot deploy because of health concerns, the ripple effect impacts our military's defense capabilities. The DoD spends an estimated $3 billion yearly on personnel costs for nondeployable Army soldiers alone.

Service members unable to deploy because of health issues cannot perform their duties, leave the military, or collect compensation until their case is resolved—a process that can take years.

Post-traumatic stress disorder remains the leading cause of service member disability, along with major depressive disorders and traumatic brain injuries. These invisible wounds affect both DoD readiness and the well-being of our troops and their families during enlistment and after their discharge. As I mentioned, approximately seventeen veterans die by suicide every day.

With capabilities enhanced by AI, MERIT could shorten the wait time for these service members with health issues by 180 days, saving the military billions of dollars.

MERIT's predictive modeling capabilities apply machine learning to create targeted, timely analytics based on the twenty-four most common service-ending disabilities. The toolset allows health professionals to assess the probability of disability trending over time. MERIT helps identify how a health issue might deteriorate and get ahead of the problem. MERIT could also help the military's health professionals improve the treatment of chronic health conditions.

What is the future of MERIT in a world where individual genomes can be sequenced? We see precision individualized medicine transforming healthcare delivery. Consistent scanning of individual patient information, monitoring behaviors, exposures, and other data can provide insights that could send alerts to protect health, improve wellness, and ultimately, extend lifespans and enhance quality of life— not just for service members but for all.

Michelle shares, "One of the great successes during COVID was that we were able to integrate seventy data sets and create twenty-six laws that allowed us to support NORAD, NORTHCOM, and the Guard Bureau during COVID."

NORAD, the North American Aerospace Defense Command, provides aerospace warning, air sovereignty, and protection for the continental United States and Canada. NORTHCOM, the US Northern Command, plans, organizes, and executes homeland defense and civil support missions. The Guard Bureau is responsible for administering the National Guard.

"We were helping identify where to focus immunizations because of increased death rates or because they were rural and didn't have access like other people," Michelle explains. "[Another thing] that we did during COVID [was] utilizing our health imaging data to predict outcomes with COVID-19 infections. In the beginning we were using chest X-rays that were a better predictor than the original test swabs—there weren't any swabs at the time. Because we had to solve for COVID, a lot came out of it. One of the things that we did was utilize our insider threat capabilities and apply them toward suicide prevention. Truly, AI has created the foundation to enable digital transformation for twenty-first-century healthcare."

While at the JAIC, Michelle also served as director of Warfighter Health Predictive Readiness Analytics. Like me, Michelle has moved on from the JAIC. She recently shared these further impressions about our times together there.

It was a unique and fun experience—and historic. At what other time in history have we changed something so significantly? I had been working with the Air Force chief of staff to stand up the Invisible Wounds Initiative,[6] which serves airmen living with PTSD and TBI (traumatic brain injury).

Part of the work was to create a support structure for the conditions in life that make us successful in protecting our national interest and our people—AI readiness, policies, infrastructure, and workforce and talent management. We were searching for a place to build an integrated treatment clinic. We also did some work in AI. When I briefed my ideas to the Undersecretary of Defense for Policy and Readiness, he said, "We are standing up a Joint Artificial Intelligence Center, and we think you need to work there." A conversation took place with General Shanahan. He told me, "Michelle, this is awesome. Nobody will argue with me about the work you're thinking about doing. And by the way, I just brought somebody else on board. His name is Hassan. I think you guys are going to work well together."

The whole team was focused on building AI success stories and then taking technology and turning it into capability for the DoD. I oversaw the capitalization of EHRs, health record analysis, and all of the cases we could come up with that we could apply to make a difference in people's health.

I wanted to expedite changes to the policy process. One of the biggest challenges with applying AI to health is the policies surrounding protecting individual health records. Congress actually mandated the institution of electronic health records, known as the Military Health System (MHS) Genesis.[7] In Veterans

Affairs, it's called the Oracle Cerner Health Record System,[8] but they're both similar systems. It was the largest electronic health record rollout in history and had twelve congressional oversight committees. They were supposed to fully deploy an electronic health record by 2023.

This idea was brewing in my mind. I'm a psychotherapist by training. Worldwide, we use insurance codes, ICD 9 or ICD 10.[9] Whenever you go to a doctor to evaluate a symptom, they use a code to describe it to an insurance company. The codes are very descriptive. I wondered, "What if we map the codes to the VA's disability ratings, which have been around since 1947, and reverse engineer the model to come up with evaluations that allow us to identify the causation of disease?"

From there, I started looking at the operational cost of disabilities for the DoD—it's more than $3 billion for 1 percent of the population. Service-related disabilities consume about eight hundred readiness days per service member, and that includes the one hundred to two hundred days to recruit and train a replacement. I realized this could have a significant impact. I asked, "How can we build a model to help us drive future readiness and predict when someone will be injured?"

When you look at the injuries across the joint warfighters, 24 percent of their medical issues are musculoskeletal, followed by mental health. We thought that we could mature AI to a point where it would impact service members' health, which is truly critical to our national security.

This use of AI is really like a check engine light in our car. We wanted to enable individuals and doctors to detect conditions that lead to degraded readiness, applying predictive maintenance principles to people. Prevention becomes the focus for any health condition.

Everybody talks about the twenty-first century as the Information Age. But I say it's becoming more accurate to call it the Intelligent Information Age because we're integrating data and AI into processes that really change how we see problems and how we find solutions.

When Michelle and I were working on MERIT, we saw the return-on-investment numbers. We saw the billions of hours the system spends and the many months or years that service members wait in limbo to get their cases adjudicated.

I've been a patient in both the civilian and military realms. But going from being an active duty officer to the ranks of the retired, having had to navigate that and having worked on the problem at the Pentagon, it hit me in a visceral way. I fully appreciated the importance of the work we were doing. Sometimes, in the abstract, it's hard to appreciate what you're doing and the impact you could have. But if we get this right one day—and the military continues to work on initiatives such as MERIT and others like it—it will be a great benefit in facilitating a journey that all service members make.

Safety and Well-Being: Project Salus

During the deadly spring of 2020, COVID-19 vaccines were not yet available, and testing was limited. Yet the United States National Guard augmented civilian health systems as they sought to predict, diagnose, and prevent the spread of the coronavirus.

In late March 2020, the JAIC began coordinating with the US Northern Command and the National Guard Bureau on Project Salus, named for the Roman goddess of safety and well-being. Our Project Salus team developed a data aggregation and fusion capability armed with AI-enabled predictive analytic and resource allocation decision tools as part of the Guard's pandemic response.

By applying AI to a predictive dashboard, Project Salus helped NORTHCOM and National Guard teams identify where critical supply chain shortages might occur. At the very beginning of March, no one knew what COVID-19 was, and we needed better testing. With the help of AI, we were able to opine when people would come down with COVID-19. We fed in data about the numbers of people engaging with hospital emergency rooms and clinics and coming in en masse showing signs of COVID-19—coughing and flu-like symptoms. We worked with our teams of engineers and analysts and partnered with the Department of Health and Human Services and the Centers for Medicare & Medicaid Services (CMS) to access their data. We used that data to build models that helped us apply these predictive algorithms.

We literally assessed more than fifteen million patient records by selecting for the ICD 10 codes—the codes Michelle referred to that healthcare personnel enter when submitting billing to insurers. These helped determine those who most likely had a COVID-19 diagnosis. And we did it without breaching patient confidentiality. Then we built models to show the hot spots where outbreaks were occurring across the United States to determine where to deploy more healthcare workers and more vaccine resources as they became available.

We were able to build out scenarios and predictions down to the zip code level. We knew where outbreaks were occurring, and we could track COVID-19 progression from community to community. Early on, we used this information to guide the deployment of resources, including personal protective equipment as well as doctors and nurses. Our public health policymakers used this information to guide and direct their instructions to the communities and the populations that were impacted.

As we got to know more and more about the disease and as testing became available, we were able to refine the models to be more predictive. By the time the vaccines were developed, we could help target areas that should be prioritized for vaccines—places where outbreaks were high and places with a lot of disease burden such as Los Angeles County and other densely populated zip codes. Initially, when vaccines were scarce, Project Salus helped direct the resources to where they were needed most. We looked at the health records of millions of people and, in this case, the claims data. With our AI models' help, we could assess which hospitals were submitting to CMS for payment and which communities were being affected by the spread of COVID-19.

This was a nice success story for us at the JAIC, a morale booster. If you remember the early part of 2020, that spring, many of us were sitting there, feeling fairly useless. We were all hunkered down at home, desperately wanting to help and assist. At the JAIC, we felt like we had to be able to do something. So we made some investments, made some decisions, and allocated resources, personnel, and expertise to the project. Early on, the folks in leadership and command relied on us to help make the decisions that formed their strategy.

This story illustrates the range of applications that an AI-enhanced health record would benefit the individual by highly personalizing preventive, diagnostic, and treatment of health conditions. It also shows how these applications would enhance the reach of our public health sectors in battling pandemics, building equity in healthcare access, and bridging gaps in services created by inefficient data management.

AHLTA VISTA and Beyond

When I was working on my Master of Public Administration at the Harvard Kennedy School of Government in 2009, I wrote a thesis examining AHLTA VISTA, the electronic medical record (EMR) systems of the Department of Veterans Affairs—Veterans Health Information Systems and Technology Architecture (VISTA)—and the Department of Defense Armed Forces Health Longitudinal Technology Application (AHLTA).

As a surgeon dealing with life and death, often making critical decisions with imperfect knowledge to achieve successful results, I wanted to improve these two EHR systems. Significant innovations, such as VISTA and AHLTA, have dramatically impacted the practice of military medicine since they were launched in 1996 and 2006. As a staff member attending cardiothoracic surgery at the DoD, National Naval Medical Center in the early 2000s, I used AHLTA almost exclusively daily.

Considerable data on the historical, quantitative, and qualitative aspects of AHLTA and VISTA can be found in the literature, particularly on VISTA, because of its longer history and use. At the time I wrote my article, costs for AHLTA and VISTA systems approached $20 billion, and combined, both systems provided EMR service for more than fourteen million military personnel, family members, veterans, and retirees—the largest EMR systems in the world.

VISTA enjoyed a positive acceptance among providers because of its ease of use, friendly graphical user interface with a computerized patient record system, and ability to provide healthcare providers with all available information in one central location. Surgeons and medical specialists appreciate being able to assess and inventory all previous tests and encounters a patient has had with their generalist physicians. This feature also allows the VA to realize a true cost-saving benefit through eliminating unnecessary testing and promoting population health through continuity of care and preventive health measures.

VISTA also had the potential to improve patient-oriented care. VA investigators from various specialties have utilized the VISTA application as a resource to establish disease-specific registries, measure and promote VA population health, improve quality and safety through risk prediction models, and promote continuity of care.

Throughout its development, AHLTA was designed to satisfy specific objectives within the DoD, not necessarily facilitate the work of the healthcare provider end user.

Both AHLTA and VISTA are incredibly successful applications. While these legacy applications should continue to provide all relevant data on individual patients and populations, what will be more essential in the future is each application's ability to intuitively provide a healthcare provider with the information necessary to treat a particular condition without the provider even searching for it. This is the hope for the next generation of EHRs.

My journey from navigating the VA system to working on the MERIT and Project Salus highlights the critical need for healthcare access and efficiency improvements for veterans and service members. My personal experiences with the VA system underscored the importance of human connection and equitable care, driving home the potential for AI to transform healthcare delivery. Through initiatives such as MERIT, which leverages AI for predictive modeling and early intervention, and Project Salus, which used AI to manage the COVID-19 response, we have demonstrated the significant impact of AI on healthcare.

These projects not only improve patient outcomes but also enhance the readiness and efficiency of our military health systems. As we integrate AI and refine EHRs, we will move closer to a future where healthcare is more personalized, accessible, and effective for all, ensuring that our service members receive the support and care they deserve. Like other medical frontiers first explored by the military, these EHR systems paved the way for parallel advances in civilian medicine. We are at the dawn of a new era and realizing great potential in the EHR data with AI.

Parallel Advances: Dr. Amol Ahmed Joshi

Dr. Amol Ahmed Joshi, Byrne Betty fellow and associate professor of strategic management and innovation and commercialization at Wake Forest University, is an affiliate faculty advisor on healthcare innovation, AI, biomedical informatics, and precision medicine. Dr. Joshi is also an experienced Silicon Valley entrepreneur who researches how inventors create and commercialize new technologies across borders.

In early 2024, Wake Forest, which has become near and dear to my heart because my son is a student there, hosted a one-day program through its School of Professional Studies on AI's emerging impact on healthcare innovation.

Healthcare professionals from a broad spectrum of viewpoints gathered to increase their understanding of making thoughtful decisions about using AI to improve patient outcomes and the performance of their organizations. Sessions highlighted research-driven approaches to AI with the latest insights from published studies and case studies, evidence-based AI medicine applications, and evidence-based AI management applications. It was really interesting to hear the different perspectives of healthcare leadership, patients, and providers.

Dr. Joshi has come full circle in his career. Trained in electrical engineering and computer engineering, he started his career designing audio products, electronics, and telecommunications technology. He founded Be Vocal, an early pioneer in speech recognition technology that could understand human speech and translate it into text that could inform intelligent business or individual decision-making.

Dr. Joshi talked about his past work in tech and current work with AI on my Forbes Books' *Smarter Healthcare with AI* podcast

When I look at where the technology is today, it is generations beyond what we even imagined. We didn't have smartphones. All our phones were docked. We didn't have the computational capabilities. We used big servers installed in phone company networks to do the kind of processing you can do on your phone right now.

That improvement in computation power has made a lot of applications possible. In the early days, it was all about reliability, getting the accuracy of the record, and recognizing the speech. We are so far beyond that today that we're finally close to reliability, where we can start credibly thinking about medical applications. The reliability threshold for a surgeon needs to be extremely high.

In working with many medical professionals at our school of medicine, the innovation is primarily software. A lot of it's the algorithm, and how does the algorithm interact with people? What is the user interface? So many advanced applications are available that I thought it was time to go back and do some fundamental research to try to help people make better decisions about how to use the technology.

Physicians have a specialized vocabulary and very precise terminology. That's actually a benefit when you're doing translation and speech recognition because you don't have to search the universe of words. There's a limited set of vocabulary that you're going to use. So we can guess ahead of time the way you will describe conditions and make a probabilistic, accurate prediction of what you might say next. The legal profession is the same way. My friends who are lawyers talk a certain way.

Using specialized, unique words actually improves the accuracy of the system. Understanding the context in which the care is provided and how the patient will interact really helps to improve these systems.

The cumulative knowledge we've gathered over the last few decades is remarkable—just amazing. Think about the content available on the internet. If you want to train search engines to recognize things, you have a huge body of content.

AI—"Why Not in Healthcare?"

If everyday people can understand how AI can be used in other areas of their lives, they will immediately say, "Why not in healthcare?" If I'm a frequent traveler and use an AI chatbot to talk to my airline, I'm very comfortable with them handling those important details and helping me. I think, "Are there other interactions where I would also be comfortable?" Maybe it's not the patient-physician interaction but certainly scheduling my next appointment or going for a lab test. The point is that the people element, the ubiquity of the technology, makes the barriers to adoption fewer, because it gives many opportunities for folks to have a trustworthy experience with AI. And I think that is really the key.

In terms of healthcare applications, I am most excited about those that allow us to detect and diagnose very serious conditions early, affecting the patient, their family, and society as a whole.

The team at Wake Forest Center for Healthcare Innovation has developed a way to analyze EHRs and use that analysis to generate a frailty score. In other words how susceptible are patients to other forms of risk? An offshoot of that research—based on the information in their healthcare records—looks at wearable devices. Are there early indicators of cognitive decline? And it actually comes full circle back to voice technology. We know that if someone's had a microstroke or earlier stroke, they could start to show signs of aphasia. These delays in word-finding can be detected and measured using the same technology we use to recognize speech.

What about taking that along with someone's gait or walking pattern? These are other indicators that you get from a wearable device—signs that something may be going wrong. These technologies are relatively within our reach and would save a lot of downstream pain and suffering and improve the lives of people worldwide.

Early detection and diagnosis of chronic conditions are going to be important areas where we could use AI. Purpose, personalization, and partnership are how to combine those technologies.

We talked about using translation or speech recognition to translate what a doctor says into medical coding. For example, you might wonder if there's an issue with how medical conditions are being coded. Are they being miscoded, undercoded, or overcoded? Ensuring this information is correct is the key part of the care process. So that's where

AI technology can be used in a way that could very much improve the experience for everyone on the caregiver, patient, and payer sides.

The First AI Application with a Billing Code

Using AI for screening diabetic retinopathy was the first autonomous AI application to have a CPT code. The FDA approved this software as a medical device. It has a Medicare billing code and is reimbursable by insurance. However, the ultimate use case for the technology was different from the original use case that the inventors had in mind.

A number of companies came together to develop autonomous AI technology to screen for diabetic retinopathy, a devastating condition that is largely preventable if detected early.

The original use case was to use this AI technology as an electronic assistant to an ophthalmologist. But ophthalmologists, highly trained specialists, didn't need it. It ended up working in clinics that didn't have an ophthalmologist and instead only had eye technicians who wanted to screen people quickly without having to dilate patients' eyes.

Medicare came in and said, "This amount of dollars is what we will pay for this." Then the clinics could figure out volume-wise how many more patients they would need to see to break even, have an effective return, and prevent downstream costs in care.

Some faculty colleagues at Wake Forest looked at this and asked, "What are the lessons learned that we can highlight?" This is one of the few areas where this reimbursement is available. So from a business point of view, I've been focused on that because, unfortunately, reimbursement is one of the big obstacles. There's a productive intersection between folks in the business world, medical providers, and health economists, each looking at it differently.

Demand Evidence in Outcomes, Cost, and Scalability

My philosophy is to be open to AI. But be cautious about the claims that are made about it. Demand evidence. Health systems, health leaders, and others considering adopting AI technology need to take a hard look at it. Are there natural experiments where data can be gathered?

Within a healthcare system, if one set of clinics has adopted a technology, what is the effect? What are the differences in the outcomes for these adoptions? Can we look at the hard data and say numerically and quantitatively that in settings that adopted this technology, it cost them this much, and that this was an observable improvement? And then what would we expect if it scales nationally?

I worry that things could be priced in an unrealistic way that skews the total cost of ownership and hides the true reality of operating the system. We have venture capital investors who are investing in these companies, who are building these technologies. There are some established companies as well, but public market investors are expecting a return and will price very aggressively.

That may hide the actual economics. The problem is that it's not like software in other areas where you can update to the cloud, and everybody gets the latest version. You need to make sure that the thing still works—look for opportunities to do these experiments, do the hardcore economic analysis, and really quantify the observable differences.

Now that's going to take time. But in a way we have time. We're dealing in a largely regulated business. Given the high level of quality that must be met, we should carefully take our time and make sure that we meet these objectives. The first rule is to do no harm.

Universities need to be proactive and actively engaged as partners in all of these things. There are three or four different areas where universities can uniquely contribute.

One, they are nonprofit institutions with a broader mission. At Wake Forest, it's *pro humanitate*, for the service of humanity. We are supposed to be working on research and ideas and training the next generation to think carefully about these different issues.

Two, there are very few other places in society where these different specialties are all under one roof—and there's not a responsibility for short-term profitability but more long-term societal impact. So we can be conveners in bringing people together from different disciplines, from engineering, sciences, medicine, ethics, cognitive psychology, and human behavior. We need to bring all those folks together.

Three, we're not just going to develop it. We'll test it on a small scale. If it's worthwhile, we'll share it. There may be a commercial aspect, but there may also be a scientific advancement aspect. We want to publish research that others can build on, cumulative knowledge. However, there may be a piece of technology that can also be licensed and shared.

Four, our other role is to be an independent, nonpartisan, and objective voice in evaluating and making recommendations at the local, state, and federal government levels—not just an opinion but some empirical evidence.

All of this together ultimately ties into our mission: training and preparing students as leaders for the future. We are training students for industries that still need to be founded in companies that have yet to be founded. The next great idea company could come from one of your medical school students who's working with a software entrepreneur and a bioethicist and comes up with a new way to do something that has a huge impact. Universities like Wake Forest and others need to play a more prominent role post-COVID as trusted advisors to society.

The thing that gives me the most optimism is our students. The young people in the generation we're working with now are digital natives. They've never known a life without the internet, without cell phones, and without technology. Not only were they born in this digital age, but they are also more global in ways that perhaps our generation or other generations were not because of connectivity. They're more aware of things that are going on around the world. They're not just looking at problems locally but thinking at a broader level. Sometimes youth and inexperience can be a great advantage.

NOTES

"Command and Control of Special Operations Forces Missions in the US Northern Command Area of Responsibility," 2005, https://core.ac.uk/download/36695929.pdf.

Takahashi, Dean, "Pocket Gems Says Mobile-Focused Game Companies Will Win, VentureBeat, May 27, 2011, https://venturebeat.com/games/pocket-gems-says-mobile-focused-game-companies-will-win/.

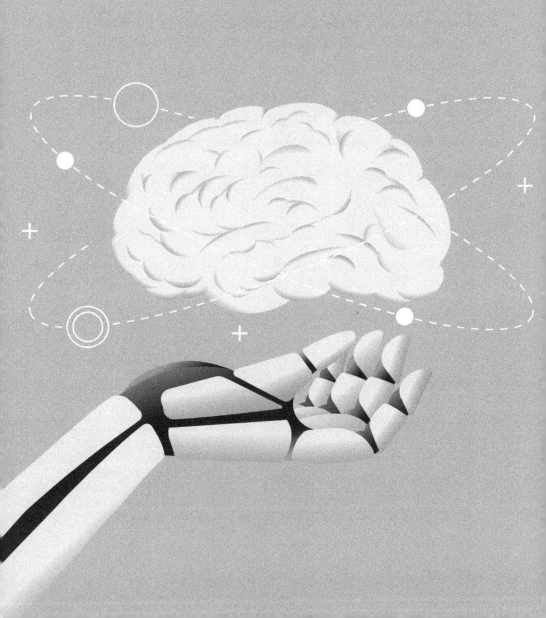

CHAPTER 5

CAN AN ALGORITHM PREVENT SUICIDE?

S uicide is the second leading cause of death in the US military. So it made sense during my tenure at the JAIC that our team researched how AI could be employed as a preventive measure. Led by Colonel Caesar Junker, USAF, leader of the Human Performance Portfolio for the team, our goal for the project was to develop an AI-enabled suicide intervention and prevention tool that could identify risk factors and alert commanders and medical providers when a service member was a high risk for death by suicide.

At the beginning of my time at the JAIC, Colonel Caesar Junker came to mind as I recruited talented, good people to work with. I had met Colonel Junker years before when I was a young lieutenant commander, and he was already my colonel. I knew him as the physician for Air Force One, among many roles. He was a great leader and my mentor.

In 2012, I worked as assistant deputy commander for the Business of Healthcare Operations Directorate at the National Naval Medical

Center during its merger with Walter Reed Medical Center. Caesar started to work with our group as part of the Air Force leadership to promote their health initiatives. I received the news that I was being transferred to Navy Medicine Headquarters to serve as health policy advisor to the Navy surgeon general under the M5 Strategy Directorate of the Bureau of Medicine and Surgery. I was hoping he could take over my role, but then he got called away as well.

So when I had the great fortune many years later to go to the JAIC, I reached out to him. He and Michelle Padgett had worked together for the Air Force Chief of Staff. Caesar was one of the people leading the Air Force Surgeon General's human performance initiative. I told him about our AI initiatives. I knew that he would be interested in our ideas for suicide prevention and human performance. Well, he came on board. And in true Colonel Junker form, he asked, "How do we make things better for our service members? How do we prevent suicide? How do we maximize their performance? And when we think about human performance, how do we address the whole person so they can be the best version of themselves mentally, spiritually, and physically?"

Never Discount the Power of a Dinner

After Caesar joined us at the JAIC, we brainstormed a lot. One day he invited me to dinner with some of his colleagues and leaders within an organization, Patients Like Me, a fascinating group of folks. This organization offers a social media forum and platform for people with chronic diseases and healthcare issues. As we all conversed, Caesar shared that the JAIC was working on ways to help service members achieve enhanced human performance and be the best version of themselves—but that they never could achieve that if they had suicidal thoughts or died by suicide. We asked our dinner partners how people on the forum addressed the challenging problems that they encountered, and they shared many good insights.

Then Caesar mentioned that in the military, when a service member dies by suicide, there is quite a bit of investigation, including interviews with friends, family, and commanders, and examinations of social media. This investigation generates a report, basically a forensic analysis of the patient's life—social, financial, professional, personal, and criminal. That report is submitted to the commanding officer for evaluation to see what might be learned. As we discussed this, we concluded that it would be interesting to see if patterns emerged within all of this information. This dinner with colleagues was the launchpad for our work to use AI to prevent suicides in the military.

That was the beginning of Project Orion. We left that dinner completely inspired. The moral of the story is never, never discount the power of a dinner, a mastermind meeting of like-minded people who want to solve a significant problem in a casual setting. Sometimes, that's where the best and most brilliant ideas originate. I recently asked Caesar to share more about Project Orion, and he offered the following:

Our goal for Project Orion was to target suicide prevention with AI initiatives. There was a lot of research and programs already using technology to improve our ability to treat those who were at high risk for suicide.

Whenever you introduce artificial intelligence, the primary goal is to accumulate data in order to train the computer to learn. In this case we used postmortem reports—basically psychological autopsies on the military individuals who had died by suicide. Unlike other organizations where only nefarious activity is ruled out and the investigation is limited, when you find out that someone was killed by suicide in the military, there's a real investigation. So a copious amount of information is collected—hundreds of pages on one patient.

We were able to start with five hundred death reports. Those reports contained interviews, pictures, videos, text messages, social media, and lots of data in all sorts of forms. From this investigation, we gained a lot of insight into why individuals died by suicide. We had the relevant information to create dashboards to help commanders in the field use the data to potentially help prevent suicides.

There are a lot of limitations any time you're using data to try to help prevent a negative event from occurring in a soldier's life. My role was to try to really look at the entire landscape of what was being done.

Our number one goal was to use algorithms that could use the data to teach AI to get better at predicting. Suicide is such a small incident rate. That makes it difficult to try to predict. So we use something called an insider threat program, where AI is used to try to predict the future and, when necessary, notify commanders and make interventions.

The biggest roadblock is always going to be privacy concerns. We must consider the risk/benefit ratio—what are the negatives and the positives? A positive is using AI to tell the healthcare provider that a person is at higher risk for some sort of mental health event so they can conclude, "Okay, we need to pay more attention to this patient."

Suicide and the Quest for Optimal Human Performance

If service members are having thoughts of harming themselves or engaging in destructive behaviors, they'll never maximize that best version of themselves. So before we even started talking about maximizing their potential and achieving optimal human performance, we had to look at suicide. The military hadn't found a good way to address it at that time despite many different initiatives. Lots of people cared about it. Lots of people gave money. Lots of leaders were concerned. And we'd all known someone, God bless, whom we had lost. I know our JAIC team did.

Suicide is a really complicated, difficult, challenging problem—one for which we don't have good answers.

Data is the food that AI needs to grow strong. And like Caesar mentioned, there is no shortage of it in the military. For suicide risk, known contributors to dangerous levels of stress can include family or relationship issues, financial difficulties, medical conditions such as chronic pain or combat injuries, substance use disorders, or past trauma on the battlefield that resulted in PTSD. That living data could be combined with data retrieved from the military's postmortem reports to create the algorithms needed for more accurate prediction of suicidal tendencies.

Caesar and I both believe that using AI to predict suicide risk would not only increase the military's readiness but also benefit each service member along with their families. And its application in the civilian world could save even more lives. In the United States, suicide is among the top nine leading causes of death for people ages ten to sixty-four—and the second leading cause of death for younger folks, ages ten to fourteen and twenty to thirty-four.[10]

Suicide rates also differ by race, ethnicity, career path, and where people live. American Indian and Alaska Native people have the highest rates of death by suicide, followed by non-Hispanic whites. People living in rural areas or working in mining and construction are also at higher risk, as are young people who identify as LGBTQ.

When the right AI algorithm is developed, it could potentially be applied to medical records, financial records, behavioral reports, and other information to identify the risk for suicide per data uploaded from those military postmortem reports.

Meanwhile, all branches of the US military have programs to help prevent suicide. The Army has employed its colossal Study to Assess Risk and Resilience in Servicemembers,[11] a massive longitudinal research study into suicide prevention. The Navy employs its Sailor Assistance and Intercept for Life program, which provides rapid assistance, regular risk assessment, and resource referral. The Marine Corps Suicide Prevention System includes a Command Suicide Prevention and Risk Mitigation Strategies publication that presents scenarios and corresponding prevention strategies. The Air Force Suicide Prevention Program launched in 1996. And the Coast Guard's Applied Suicide Intervention Skills Training enlists peer supports.

Even so, a study compiling data from 2001 through 2009 found that 21.3 percent of deployed service members' deaths during the Iraq and Afghanistan wars were due to suicide. And 19.7 percent of deaths of Iraq and Afghanistan war veterans were deaths by suicide.[12]

AI Could Reduce Those Numbers

While the JAIC's AI-enabled Suicide Intervention and Prevention tool was embryonic, hopes are that some aspects of it will someday be utilized and deployed in the future to address this significant problem. As part of a data-driven composite display of behavioral risks, the Commanders' Risk Mitigation Dashboard will improve a leader's situational awareness of crewmembers at risk for a variety of destructive behaviors, including suicide. Commanders will have the information they need to make interventions. By applying an AI algorithm to DHA Medical Records, the military's EHR system could alert military medical providers when a patient is at risk for suicide.

In 2021, while I was still leading the JAIC's health mission, Allan Ripp from the *Wall Street Journal*[13] gave me a call. It can be quite a surprise to learn how others perceive you, but when he wrote that I was "an unabashed medical nerd," I didn't mind because he went on to quote me as I explained why I believed advancing the use of AI in healthcare was essential not only to warfighter health but also to our nation's security. I said, "What the X-ray or anesthesia were to medicine generations ago, AI is today in its essentiality. You can call me an evangelist, a proselytizer, or a broken record—it's all fine. Vladimir Putin had it right when he predicted whichever nation leads in artificial intelligence will dominate. In the arms race for healthcare AI, I want to make sure the United States doesn't come in second."

Well, suicide is coming in second—the second leading cause of death for our service members. Suicide is also the second leading cause of death for our brave veterans.[14] And in the civilian sector, suicide is the second leading cause of death among our children ages ten to fourteen and young adults ages twenty to thirty-four.[15] Think about that. Only accidents kill more of our ten-year-olds than suicide.[16] How can we, as a nation, as a military force, come in first when suicide is our second leading cause of death?

In chapter 2, we talked about how the US military has driven many medical advances. With the help of AI, it can drive the advancement of suicide prevention as well. I do not suggest AI is a panacea. However, AI could provide care providers and individuals with the predictive technology to deliver help to those in need before that ten-year-old, that young service member, or that decorated veteran takes their own life.

As I told Allan Ripp, today's big breakthroughs come from harnessing information, which can be provided by the military's massive computing power and those robust "lust to dust" EHRs. By the way, that medical imaging portfolio across the Defense Department houses hundreds of millions of images—CT scans, MRIs, X-rays. When I was at the JAIC, we created algorithms from some of this portfolio to help improve diagnoses and to research new therapeutics, an endeavor akin to the human genome project in scale and long-term importance. As I mentioned we also sought to collaborate with the JPC, a repository of millions of tissue specimens the military has collected for over one hundred years. And don't forget, the military has detailed forensic reports on every service member who died by suicide.

With the assistance of behavioral experts at Harvard and Johns Hopkins, our Project Orion team applied AI to use natural language processing to detect patterns and outlier events across those report documents to identify societal, emotional, and other triggers that took the service person to the edge. Our effort gleaned trends, including many unobvious ones, which could pick up signals for suicide ideation or high-risk behavior by future service members that could be flagged for military commanders and medical providers. It may sound grandiose, but Orion was about ontology (the nature of being), context, and the totality of a person's existence.

With the data sources available today—data sources that are multiplying exponentially—what we learned in Project Orion could be applied to the civilian sector. We could require our public health institutions to collect more data on individuals who die by suicide.

We could develop ways to harvest data from social media that goes beyond flagging us for an ad for a product to giving us help with mental health resources—and alerting local mental health crisis care professionals. Yes, privacy will be an issue. But with the power of AI, we can certainly find a way to *protect both* privacy and save lives.

AI at Its Apogee

AI has evolved a lot, which is why it is at the forefront of everyone's mind. It was described decades ago, but no one was talking about it. Those of us who have been in this space for years see this as a novel time, a critical space that has brought AI to the apogee, this zeitgeist where everyone knows about it, talks about it, and is fearful of it.

We now have the capacity to exchange information at a pace that we never had before. In the past we faxed documents back and forth. Now you can attach a one-thousand-page PDF and send it on your phone. We have a lot more data. We have computing power we didn't have before. We have a network of connectivity. We have really bright people developing algorithms, developing technology, and building the infrastructure to make AI a lot more effective, visible, and impactful.

AI will impact everything. I'm going to repeat that. AI will impact *everything*, except for the things that matter most. If it wasn't for electricity, you and I could still exchange ideas in the dark, sitting by candlelight. The crux of what matters is your relationships, caring for your family, and taking care of yourself; those things will still happen with or without AI.

However, now you can use AI to leverage those interactions to improve care, education, and fitness and potentially prevent suicide. Let's regard AI for what it is: a tool, a technology, an innovation that undoubtedly impacts every aspect of our lives. As I mentioned, suicide

SMARTER HEALTHCARE WITH AI

is the second leading cause of death for service members, veterans, and young people. The incidence of suicide is also rising among older adults—men aged seventy-five and older have the highest overall rate of suicide. We have identified a problem. We also have a tool called AI and data analysis technology. We can apply these innovations to address this problem, right?

I would encourage everyone not to think of technology as amorphous or ambiguous. Like all tools, whether it's good, bad, or evil depends on who uses it. And we can use this tool, this technology to do something good—decrease the incidence of suicide.

I am a runner. I've completed twenty-five marathons, and in 2024 I completed my first Ironman 70.3. In conversations with my running and triathlon peers, I hear them talk about how AI has helped them develop running plans, diets, and other ways to meet their fitness goals. AI could also help people meet their mental health goals.

While I understand people are nervous about ChatGPT, what if AI tools such as this could be utilized to talk down people from the ledge? By accessing that person's data, it could come up with a personalized dialogue with the right words and the right motivation to spark that glimmer of hope that could help that person. Now of course, we may not want a robot delivering that dialogue. But the first responder on the scene could be instantly coached with the right words to say.

One of the things I used to love doing was going into a music store, such as Tower Records in New York City, and looking at records. (It closed in 2006.) It was one of those iconic places before streaming music became the norm. That was one of my favorite pastimes. When I moved to DC in 2009, I wanted to hear a certain song. Foolishly, I got into my car and drove to the mall. I walked through the entire mall, but there was no music store. I thought, "How is this possible?"

It had been a while since I'd gone out to buy music because I had a pretty good collection. That's when it dawned on me that I had not fully embraced a change that happened, an evolution. I figured out how to download music. But that experience reinforced what I'm trying to convey. Don't be the one who gets into the car in 2009 and drives to the mall to try to find a CD.

Today, music stores are back. Vinyl is back. Tower Records reopened in 2023 as Tower Labs, which aims to create space for performers to socialize before and after shows. We can stream our music and hold it in our own hands too. We can have both the familiar personal and the abstract technical. Both the hands-on and the virtual connection to a patient. Indeed, we can confidentially and ethically access vast amounts of data that can point us to someone needing help.

In June 2023 this headline appeared in Stat News,[17] which delivers journalism about health, medicine, and the life sciences: "A 988 operator, faced with a flood of calls, turns to AI to boost counselor skills." The article goes on to share how, in Portland, Oregon, more than one thousand 988 Suicide & Crisis Lifeline calls were coming in. Concerns were mounting that, though thoroughly trained, counselors would potentially fail to handle calls from people at imminent risk of suicide.

Protocall, the company handling the call tech for 988 in Portland, sought out Lyssn. This company had developed a platform that uses AI to analyze and review recordings of behavioral health encounters. A $2 million grant from the National Institute of Mental Health is helping Protocol and Lyssn to adapt the tech for use in crisis calls.

Since 988's inception in 2022, the Lifeline has received more than twenty million calls from people in crisis. With numbers like those, how can we not use AI to prevent suicide?

NOTES

"An Attempted Suicide with Kelsey Lewis," *Ordinary People, Extraordinary Things*, February 13, 2023, https://www.buzzsprout.com/1882033/12231876-37-an-attempted-suicide-with-kelsey-lewis.

"A First-in-the-Nation 988 Line for Native People Goes Live in WA," NNED, March 6, 2023, https://nned.net/11803/.

"Technology (Knowledge)," Hasten the Day, https://www.hastentheday.info/technology-knowledge-transportation.

"Children and Suicide: Grief, Pain and Anguish," Work Smart Live Smart, September 10, https://worksmartlivesmart.com/stop-a-suicide-day-september/.

"A 988 Operator, Faced with a Flood of Calls, Turns to AI to Boost Counselor Skills," STAT News, June 22, 2023, https://www.thermalpr.com/news/a-988-operator-faced-with-a-flood-of-calls-turns-to-ai-to-boost-counselor-skills/.

"Do You Get the Winter Blah's? Light Therapy Might Not Be the Best Treatment," EarthScape, November 5, 2015, http://www.earthscape.org/science/news/do-you-get-the-winter-blahs-light-therapy-might-not-be-the-best-treatment/.

"Hotline Archives," RISQ Consulting, https://risqconsulting.com/tag/hotline/.

CHAPTER 6

POINT-OF-INJURY TREATMENT SUPPORT

Little did I know that my path to clinical informatics and AI would begin in the desert. As he shares here, my friend, colleague, and fellow Navy surgeon Dr. Christopher Dewing has never forgotten our first days together in Afghanistan.

> It took over ten days and a combination of civilian and military aircraft to get our surgical unit to its assigned forward operating base, to its particularly "kinetic" corner of the Helmand River Valley of Southwest Afghanistan. We clambered out of the belly of our massive transport helicopter, struggling under the weight of our combat gear, onto the rocky airfield and dragged our bags toward the medical tents, just visible over the HESCO barriers. We were all cursing the blistering heat and dust—and the fact that no

one had come out to give us a hand with our gear—when we saw the Army DUSTOFF helicopters coming onto the base low and fast.

The existing Navy surgical team, which we had come to replace, cleared us to the side. Their corpsmen sprinted out to the Blackhawks and came back carrying a limp and mangled body. The Marine's legs were gone, and what was left of his thighs was beyond recognition, a tangle of ripped, burned, bloody muscle and bone. We stood there, frozen for that split second, by shock, horror, and fear. Then abruptly the Marine sat bolt upright and glared at us before collapsing into unconsciousness as he was rushed into the tent. Hassan and I struggled out of our flak jackets and Kevlar helmets and pushed inside.

I will never forget our "operating room," an old, sagging GP tent with just enough space to accommodate one litter stand, an anesthesia machine, and basic surgical equipment. No matter how much we cleaned it, dust found its way into and onto everything. With all the lights on, it still felt dark, and the temperature rarely dipped below one hundred degrees. Our patients came to us straight from the battlefield, in severe shock from the massive blood loss of multiple amputations.

We operated, two surgeons on each side of the table, in a race to definitively control bleeding. The anesthesia team used rapid infusers to replace volume, often using fresh, whole blood from a "walking blood bank" of Marines and soldiers, eager to help us by donating their own blood on the spot.

The urgency and austerity of the surgery was a shock to all of us, but especially to Hassan, whose cardiothoracic training and practice emphasized elegance, precision, and technical perfection. After a few cases, we all accepted battlefield surgery's brutality and frugality. We had no choice; lives were hanging in the balance. We focused on cheating death. We counted on each other and clung to our faith. We never lost a patient in the tent. If they came in with a pulse, they left stable and strong enough to begin the many stages of their medevac homeward.

Some patients died just before the courageous Army DUSTOFF crews could get them to us. We tried everything we could to bring them back. Hassan opened their chests, guiding us through cardiac massage and advanced resuscitation. But their wounds and blood loss were nonsurvivable. Our "hero" patients were meticulously prepared, and their bodies were draped with our ensign. We all lined the honor guard procession from the tent to the flight line, standing at attention until the helicopters lifted away to the south.

In between cases, we fought off the anxiety and anticipation of the next trauma arrival with exercise, conversation, reading, and prayer. Access to the internet was limited, so Hassan and I leased a small satellite system from a British vendor at the closest big base and spent the better part of a week crawling around on top of the quad containers behind our medical tents, running cable, tracking satellites, and tuning our dish. Our Wi-Fi was a huge morale booster for the whole medical team.

Point-of-Injury Support, the Ultimate Lifesaver

One problem militaries have faced since the inception of war is point-of-injury support, which is military jargon for providing lifesaving treatment to warfighters who've been seriously wounded in battle.

Point-of-injury care on the battlefield has come a long way since the military stood up MASH tents during the Korean War. While the "golden hour" once was the standard, by 2009 medics serving in the US wars in Iraq and Afghanistan were focusing on the "platinum minutes," the first ten minutes when they controlled bleeding with more effective tourniquets and arranged rapid evacuation, making what were once deadly injuries survivable. The most seriously injured warfighters receive specialized care within twenty-four to forty-eight hours after combat injuries.

In addition, stationing trauma specialists closer to the battlefield and providing telemedicine access to other specialists at military hospitals have contributed to the best hospital survivability rates recorded in armed conflict. By July 2010 more than ten thousand military medical personnel were deployed to Iraq and Afghanistan.

Guiding all these efforts, a specialized patient database, the Joint Theater Trauma Registry, provides minute-by-minute data that reduces evacuation times.

In a February 2010 report, the Government Accountability Office stated, "Conducting counterinsurgency operations in often uncertain, dangerous environments such as Iraq and Afghanistan, Army theater commanders have reconfigured the composition of field hospitals and forward surgical teams by breaking them down into smaller, stand-alone units to better position them to give the severely wounded or injured—such as the casualties of blast-type injuries—the advanced emergency medical care needed to save lives."[18]

AI and Point-of-Injury Care

During my tenure at the JAIC, we examined a series of AI models that could enhance the ability to prevent, identify, and provide point-of-injury treatment support, which is essential for maintaining warfighter health and readiness.

AI could assess and analyze a wounded individual's military health records and instantly prescribe the best emergency care treatment plan, dispatch type-matched blood via drone, and coordinate transport to the facility best suited for treatment. Once the emergency has passed, AI could evaluate elements of the service member's service record and deployments to predict how likely they are to be medically boarded out of the military. That predictive analysis can be overlaid on a case to expedite the person's adjudication. This allows the service member to get their disposition faster and learn sooner whether they'll need to alter their career path.

While the standard way to respond to seriously wounded warfighters at the point of injury is to send in a helicopter to evacuate them to care away from the battlefield, studies have introduced the idea of sending the surgical team to the warfighter.[19] AI could guide these teams. At some point in the future, drones may be deployed to assess casualties, and robots may be employed to triage and stabilize the wounded warrior. These technologies may work in concert to then transport the wounded warrior to the medical unit or hospital most suited to continue their care.

AI is already being employed for point-of-injury care in the civilian world. For example, algorithms are being used to predict the severity of motor vehicle crashes, which can help inform emergency responses.[20] Once on the scene, AI can help emergency services triage patients remotely to inform transfer location and urgency.

AI-Enhanced Medical Care on the Battlefield

The care a seriously injured person receives at the point of injury has a great influence on whether they will survive and what their quality of life will be if they do. In the military approximately 90 percent of combat-related deaths occur before the patient reaches a medical treatment facility.[21] In addition, when warfighters are evacuated or engaged in providing care for others, the unit cannot complete its mission.

Trauma deaths are typically classified into three categories: immediate, early, and late.[22] Immediate deaths occur within seconds to minutes of injury and are generally unpreventable. These might include high spinal injury, brain injury, or catastrophic hemorrhage. Early deaths occur within minutes to hours after injury and are typically hemorrhage related. Late deaths occur days to weeks after injury. Had those succumbing to these late deaths received adequate care within the "golden hour," many would have survived. When the caregivers who are available at the point of injury are not proficiently trained or lack the resources to treat these wounded warfighters, their conditions are often complicated by pain, inflammation, infection, organ dysfunction, and death over days to weeks.

Despite the complexity of injuries, prehospital care is almost always immediately provided by the warfighters themselves or a buddy aid. A medic or corpsman lead team follows up and stabilizes the casualty for evacuation. A study of the 75th Ranger Regiment during Operation Enduring Freedom found that nonmedical personnel with minimal medical training[23] performed hemorrhage control interventions on 26 percent of the 419 casualties. In other words approximately 110 wounded service members—or their buddies— were the ones trying to stop life-threatening loss of blood.

AI-enhanced technology could extend the capabilities of these wounded warriors and their buddies. It could also increase the capacity of each military operation's healthcare system.[24] However, because of the extreme and unique nature of military prehospital care, technological advancements in health-related AI, machine learning, and robotics have already saved lives in the commercial sector but have yet to be successfully translated into military trauma care. Certainly, collecting data is a challenge. This may be the one instance when military medicine is not leading the development of innovative, lifesaving treatments. It is very challenging to design technology for use on the battlefield.

Given the number of constraints and our need to understand how care is provided in these contexts, it is difficult to design technology for use on the battlefield. Here, nonexpert physicians deal with extreme polytrauma cases, have limited resources, and often lack appropriate medical equipment. Data is lacking too. Less than 10 percent of care in these contexts has documentation, none of which is completed in real time.[25]

To succeed, technology for prehospital and prolonged field care on the battlefield must be small, lightweight, inexpensive, nonbreakable, easily replaceable, and have minimal power requirements. In addition, it must provide online connectivity off the network and cybersecurity. These technologies must be simple to use with intuitive interaction and have an extremely low failure rate.

To build the needed medical robotics, predictive AI algorithms, clinical decision support systems, and autonomous casualty care, access to high-quality, multimodal, indexed, curated, and standardized datasets will be required—datasets that provide pertinent context, have been annotated with real-time data, and are housed in a common environment that fosters collaborative innovation.

The TRUMAN Prehospital Data Commons

During my time at the JAIC, the DoD prioritized researching and developing Medical Robotics and Autonomous Systems to augment and scale trauma care delivery. Through its ability to train and learn on many use cases involving combat-related injuries and treatments, AI showed particular promise for providing this augmented decision support system to medically trained and untrained personnel. AI could make possible predictive diagnostic algorithms, computer-aided treatment decisions, medical robotics, closed-loop critical care, unmanned medical evacuations, and improved medical data collection and synchronization.

Our solution was the TRaUma Medical AssistaNt (TRUMAN) Prehospital Data Commons. While working with Colonel Jeremy Pamplin and his team at the Army's Telemedicine and Advanced Technology Research Center, we believed the TRUMAN Data Commons would bring us to a future where the best possible combat casualty care was AI enabled.

The TRUMAN Prehospital Data Commons initiative sought to unify relevant military and civilian prehospital data into a common location to develop AI and machine learning. The goal was to improve survivability of life, limb, and quality of life for injured warfighters. The data commons would provide storage and management of well-curated, annotated, but disparate data collected during care in military-specific medical simulation and training events and from relevant civilian data recorded during real patient care.

The data could include time series and discrete physiological data, video feeds, images, machine-readable documentation, handwritten documentation, audio files, medical records, geographic information, and environmental and contextual information. Once implemented, the Prehospital Data Commons would serve as the central location for up-to-date information on cutting-edge research and development efforts.

TRUMAN OVERVIEW

AI-driven simulation tools for training military medical personnel

AI-driven diagnostic tools at the injury site

Remote monitoring of vital signs and telementoring by remote experts

AI in treatment decision-making

Automated and robot-assisted medical procedures

The Prehospital Data Commons would include data harmonization, reusable data and AI tools, and computer resources developed specifically to support prehospital research. We proposed that the Joint Common Foundation of the JAIC would provide storage, processing capabilities, and foundational machine learning and AI tools. The platform would provide researchers and developers in the military, government, academia, and industry secure and appropriate access to the Prehospital Data Commons as necessary in order to continue adapting current technologies for military use while developing new and innovative strategies targeted at uniquely military issues.

As the TRUMAN initiative progressed, we engaged stakeholders to brainstorm technology challenges and policy concerns—data governance, common data standards, and working with personally identifiable information and classified data. We interviewed researchers, practitioners, and advanced developers. We completed an extensive review of current research and development within the field to fully incorporate the needs of the prehospital community and gather input from the medical, operational, and other relevant staff in those prehospital communities.

By providing researchers with access to a centralized database in a controlled, accessible, and secure environment and sharing capabilities such as data harmonization, reusable data science, and AI tools, we hoped that researchers and developers would be able to adapt emerging technologies for military applications and develop new technologies to improve the military prehospital environment. We saw the Prehospital Data Commons as a prerequisite to accelerating the delivery of AI and machine learning to the military medicine space and, as a result, keeping more wounded warriors alive, reducing the number of unnecessary medical evacuations, improving their quality of life after injury, and increasing the number of re-deployable warfighters.

AI Algorithm Assesses Hemorrhage Risk and Guides Treatment

Hemorrhage remains the leading cause of death on the battlefield. In fact, 91 percent of potentially survivable deaths on the battlefield are caused by hemorrhage. Data from the recent conflicts in Iraq and Afghanistan suggest that up to 24 percent of injured soldiers who bled to death before reaching a military medical treatment facility could have survived if they had been quickly identified and treated.

US Army Medical Research and Development Command's Biotechnology High-Performance Computing Software Applications Institute (BHSAI), led by Dr. Jaques Reifman, developed an AI-powered smartphone app to assess trauma patients' risk of hemorrhage. This AI-guided app, Automated Processing of the

Physiological Registry for Assessment of Injury Severity-Hemorrhage Risk Index (APPRAISE-HRI), uses an algorithm along with vital sign data such as heart rate and blood pressure from Bluetooth-connected monitors to rapidly predict the likelihood of uncontrolled bleeding. Cleared by the FDA, it is the first triage system of its kind authorized to evaluate hemorrhage risks in trauma patients. This FDA clearance marks a significant technological and regulatory milestone and opens pathways for the application's commercial licensing, aiming to make this lifesaving technology widely available.

APPRAISE-HRI could help medics on the front line by providing accurate, data-driven information through predictive analytics. It could stratify hemorrhage risks within ten minutes, potentially saving lives by enabling timely and informed medical interventions.

APPRAISE-HRI's algorithms are geared toward two levels of care. One, for those providing the first medical care that military personnel receive with the goals of either returning the service member to duty or arranging a speedy evacuation to care, and two, for advanced trauma management and emergency medical treatment during transport to level 1 trauma centers. The research team demonstrated that the APPRAISE algorithm could notify patients at risk for hemorrhage within the first ten minutes of transport and more than twenty minutes before arrival at a trauma center.

APPRAISE–HRI identifies injured soldiers at greatest risk of hemorrhage using an AI-based linear regression model that stratifies hemorrhage risk into low (HRI:I), average (HRI:II), and high (HRI:III). After training and testing the algorithm, the team compiled 540 hours of continuous vital sign data collected from 1,659 trauma patients before they got to the hospital and emergency department.

The trial's results found that the APPRAISE-HRI algorithm created a new capability to evaluate routine vital signs and alert medics to specific casualties with the highest risk of hemorrhage, thus optimizing decision-making for triage, treatment, and evacuation.

Of course, the use of algorithms such as APPRAISE-HRI has implications for the civilian population as well. With firearms contributing to more deaths among US children and teens than any other injury or illness, predicting hemorrhage could save many of those lives.[26] Gunshot wounds are also the leading cause of death among American adults. Internal bleeding is also a leading cause of death in Americans under forty-six after a car accident.[27] Worldwide, hemorrhage is the leading cause of maternal mortality, accounting for 27 percent of all maternal deaths—and 11.2 percent of maternal deaths in the United States.[28] If first responders were able to access an AI-guided algorithm such as APPRAISE-HRI, many of these lives could be saved by providing information to care providers to prepare adequately for resuscitation of injured individuals.

Dr. Reifman's journey, from the idea's inception to FDA approval and recognition with a Service to America Medal, underscores the profound impact that dedicated research and development in military healthcare can achieve. This case exemplifies how AI can be harnessed to enhance trauma care, offering a crucial tool in the medical response to injuries both on the battlefield and in civilian emergencies.

CHAPTER 6

NOTES

Gellerfors, M., Linde, J., and Gryth, D., "Helicopter In-flight Resuscitation with Freeze-Dried Plasma of a Patient with a High-Velocity Gunshot Wound to the Neck in Afghanistan—a Case Report," *Prehospital and Disaster Medicine* 30, no. 5 (2015), https://doi.org/10.1017/s1049023x15005014.

Publication, USDA ARS, https://www.ars.usda.gov/research/publications/publication/?seqNo115=228333.

Stallings, J. D., Laxminarayan, S., Yu, C., Kapela, A., Frock, A., Andrew, P., Reisner, A., and Reifman, J., "APPRAISE-HRI: An Artificial Intelligence Algorithm for Triage of Hemorrhage Casualties," Wolters Kluwer Health, Inc., *Shock* (2023), https://doi.org/10.1097/shk.0000000000002166.

"Switzerland: WHO Announces the First Meeting of the Postpartum Hemorrhage (PPH) Bundle Guideline Development Subgroup," MENA Report (2023).

Tetteh, Hassan A., *Gifts of the Heart* (United Kingdom: eBookit.com, 2013).

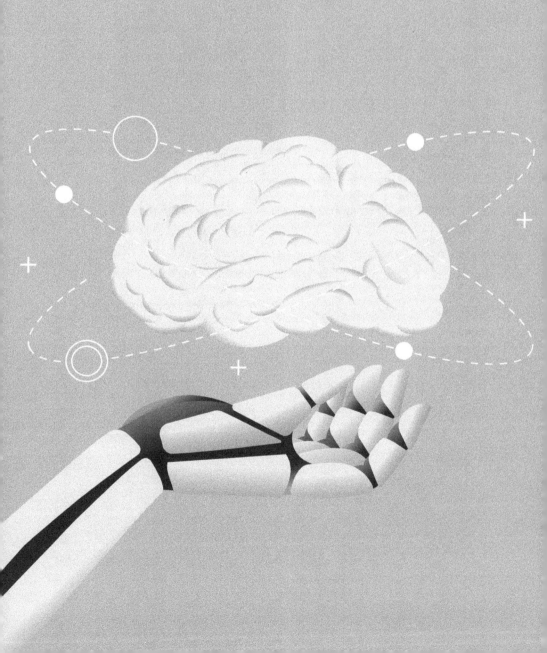

CHAPTER 7

OPERATIONALIZING ETHICS IN HEALTHCARE: WHY DATA DIVERSITY MATTERS

The US military, often lauded as the epitome of diversity, equity, and inclusion, meticulously cultivates a reflection of US society within its ranks. This deliberate act is not merely symbolic. Instead, it's a strategic imperative. Without a diverse representation mirroring society, the organization would face blind spots, rendering it vulnerable in defending national security.

Similar meticulousness is paramount in healthcare, especially in the age of AI. The burgeoning integration of AI into healthcare systems promises groundbreaking advancements. Yet it also unveils a stark reality—disparities in healthcare persist and could even exacerbate because of biased data inputs. AI has the potential to both amplify disparities and improve health equity.

Unveiling Disparities in Healthcare

We hold these truths to be self-evident,
that all men are created equal ...
—THOMAS JEFFERSON

Soon after arriving at my first duty assignment as a thoracic surgeon at the National Naval Medical Center, I was reminded of societal disparities. A seemingly innocuous encounter in a hospital hallway shattered my moment of professional triumph. Draped in my crisp white coat emblazoned with "Hassan A. Tetteh, MD Cardiac Surgery," I had just delivered news of a successful open-heart surgery to a patient's family.

As I strode back to my office, my euphoria was abruptly punctured by a request from a white woman to clean up a spill she had created while vending a beverage. In her eyes I was not a distinguished surgeon but a Black man, presumed to be the janitor. This jarring experience encapsulates the persistent challenges of racial prejudice. It underscores the imperative for equitable healthcare practices, particularly in the age of AI, where data and bias could enter into model development, with consequences on individual and population health.

The Intersection of AI and Healthcare Disparities

Healthcare disparities reverberate globally, with recent pandemics underscoring the interconnectedness of health outcomes and social determinants of health. However, AI's promise of revolutionizing healthcare is hindered by the very data it relies upon. AI algorithms, often trained on disparate datasets, risk perpetuating and amplifying existing biases. As AI-driven solutions increase, certifying these algorithms to ensure a lack of bias—akin to safety checks for appliances or cars—becomes imperative. This certification process would necessitate rigorous vetting of data sources to ensure efficacy, equity, and unbiased outcomes.

Operationalizing Ethics in AI-Driven Healthcare

In the quest to operationalize ethics within AI-driven healthcare, the principles of *The Art of Human Care* offer a guiding framework. Purpose, personalization, and partnerships emerge as pillars for navigating complex ethical terrain while leveraging AI's transformative potential.

1. **Purpose:** Defining the Ethical Framework

   At the core of ethical healthcare lies a clear, mission-driven purpose. AI serves as a potent tool in aligning decision-making processes with organizational values. By embedding ethical guidelines into AI algorithms, healthcare providers can ensure decisions prioritize patient outcomes and equity, upholding the fundamental purpose of compassionate care delivery.

   The purpose-driven approach transcends organizational mandates, encompassing societal obligations to promote health equity. Ethical AI design must align with this broader purpose, addressing systemic biases and disparities in healthcare systems. By prioritizing fairness and inclusivity, AI technologies can catalyze transformative change, fostering a healthcare landscape where everyone receives equitable access to quality care.

2. **Personalization:** AI-Enhanced Patient-Centric Ethics

Personalization lies at the heart of patient-centric care, and AI offers unprecedented capabilities in tailoring treatments to individual needs. With individual data sovereignty, AI can deliver personalized care recommendations that transcend demographic disparities by harnessing vast patient datasets. This approach enhances treatment effectiveness and respects patient autonomy, aligning with ethical principles of beneficence and nonmaleficence.

The ethos of personalization extends beyond clinical interventions, encompassing holistic care that considers socioeconomic factors, cultural backgrounds, and individual preferences. AI-driven predictive analytics can empower healthcare providers to deliver tailored interventions that address underlying health determinants, fostering trust and engagement among diverse patient populations. AI technologies may facilitate a paradigm shift toward patient-centered healthcare through personalized care pathways, where individual needs and aspirations are paramount and care is more personalized.

3. **Partnerships:** Collaborative Ethical Decision-Making

The partnership ethos underscores the importance of collaborative relationships across the healthcare ecosystem. In our connected world, AI can catalyze fostering partnerships by facilitating data sharing and communication among stakeholders. By integrating diverse perspectives into ethical decision-making processes, AI can ensure decisions are informed, transparent, and reflective of broader societal values.

Effective partnerships transcend traditional boundaries, forging alliances between healthcare providers, patients, policymakers, industry, and community stakeholders. AI technologies and the platforms that support them are pivotal in bridging these diverse entities and enabling collective action toward common goals. Through collaborative data governance frameworks, AI can foster trust and transparency, ensuring equitable distribution of resources and opportunities within healthcare systems. By leveraging the collective wisdom of stakeholders, AI-driven partnerships may pave the way for inclusive, resilient healthcare ecosystems that prioritize equity and social justice.

It was Goethe who espoused that knowing is not enough; we must apply. Willing is not enough; we must do. Indeed, operationalizing ethics in our new AI-driven healthcare ecosystem will require more than knowing what to do. We will have to apply knowledge and have a bias for action.

Ethical AI Design via Dynamic Ethical Frameworks

In a candid interview with me, Dr. James Cimino, a renowned expert in biomedical informatics, emphasized the critical importance of ethical AI design in healthcare. Dr. Cimino underscored the need for AI systems to align with legal standards and nuanced ethical considerations. Ethical AI design lays the foundation for equitable healthcare practices by prioritizing fairness, transparency, and inclusivity.

Design thinking is applied in many fields. Ethical AI design in healthcare may be applied through a DEEDS framework—a framework that promotes Dynamic, Enhanced, Ethical Decision Support.

The application of knowledge and strategic actions is imperative to operationalizing ethics in AI-driven healthcare. In the context of integrating *The Art of Human Care Theory* with a DEEDS framework, a deed is an intentional act, particularly one of significant positive impact, driven by ethical principles and aimed at advancing the well-being of individuals within the healthcare ecosystem. A deed transcends mere action. It embodies a commitment to moral excellence, compassion, and equity, catalyzing transformative change in healthcare delivery.

To operationalize ethics in AI-driven healthcare, strategic actions must embody the principles of the DEEDS framework, empowering healthcare organizations to navigate complex ethical landscapes with purpose and precision.

Dynamic ethical frameworks serve as the cornerstone of ethical decision-making in healthcare. By harnessing the power of AI, healthcare organizations can continually refine and adapt ethical guidelines to evolving challenges and technologies. Dynamic frameworks embrace agility and responsiveness, enabling proactive responses to emerging ethical dilemmas while fostering resilience and foresight. Through iterative refinement, healthcare organizations can ensure that ethical principles remain relevant and effective in a rapidly changing landscape, upholding the highest ethical standards and promoting equitable healthcare outcomes.

Dynamic ethical frameworks represent a progressive approach to ethical decision-making in healthcare. They integrate classic ethical theories espoused by ethicists with contemporary challenges posed by AI-driven technologies. Healthcare organizations can develop robust frameworks that adapt to evolving ethical landscapes with agility and precision by incorporating principles from consequentialism, deontology, virtue ethics, and principlism—an established approach in biomedical ethics based on a set of values that medical professionals can refer to in the case of confusion or conflict.

Consequentialism posits that the morality of an action is determined by its consequences, with the greatest good for the greatest number being the ultimate goal. In AI-driven healthcare, consequentialist principles prioritize outcomes that maximize patient well-being and minimize harm. Dynamic ethical frameworks leverage AI to analyze vast datasets and predict potential outcomes, enabling healthcare organizations to proactively identify interventions that optimize health outcomes for diverse patient populations. By continually evaluating the consequences of AI-driven interventions, healthcare organizations can refine ethical guidelines to ensure they align with the principles of consequentialism and promote equitable healthcare outcomes.

Ethics: Making the Right Healthcare Decision

Deontological ethics emphasizes the importance of following moral rules and duties regardless of the consequences. I'm reminded of a recent patient who presented to the emergency department unresponsive after a fall with a devastating head injury. The trauma team that received her in the trauma bay heroically stabilized the patient.

Within hours, she was in the OR for an emergency craniotomy to evacuate the bleeding in her head. The effort was futile, and she returned to the ICU. We later learned from her next of kin that our patient had a legal and recent advanced directive with specific instructions not to initiate any measures beyond comfort care should she have a fatal injury. Could a better system of information sharing, communication, and digital sovereignty facilitated by AI have better informed the team's action upon her arrival to the emergency department? Perhaps.

In healthcare, deontological principles guide ethical decision-making by prioritizing respect for autonomy, beneficence, and nonmaleficence. Dynamic ethical frameworks integrate deontological principles into AI-driven healthcare systems by ensuring that algorithms and decision support tools adhere to both ethical guidelines and regulatory standards. By embedding deontological principles into AI design and development processes, healthcare organizations can uphold the highest standards of ethical conduct and promote patient-centered care that respects individual rights and autonomy.

Virtue ethics focuses on individuals' character traits and moral virtues, emphasizing the importance of cultivating virtuous behavior in ethical decision-making. In healthcare, virtue ethics guides practitioners to embody virtues such as compassion, empathy, and integrity in their interactions with patients and colleagues. Dynamic ethical frameworks promote virtue ethics by fostering a culture of ethical excellence within healthcare organizations. By utilizing AI-driven simulations and training programs, healthcare providers can develop the virtuous character traits necessary to navigate complex ethical dilemmas with compassion and integrity. Perhaps AI could be used to perform the mundane tasks of charting and medication reconciliation, freeing more time for personal connection between healthcare professionals and their patients. By cultivating virtuous behavior among healthcare professionals, dynamic ethical frameworks ensure that principles of ethical excellence and human flourishing guide AI-driven healthcare delivery.

As articulated by Beauchamp and Childress[29], principlism proposes four ethical principles—autonomy, beneficence, nonmaleficence, and justice—as foundational to ethical decision-making in healthcare. In

AI-driven healthcare, principlism provides a framework for evaluating the ethical implications of AI algorithms and decision support tools.

Dynamic ethical frameworks integrate principlism by ensuring that AI systems prioritize patient autonomy, promote beneficence and nonmaleficence, and uphold principles of justice and equity. By aligning AI-driven healthcare practices with the core principles of principlism, healthcare organizations can navigate complex ethical landscapes with clarity and coherence, promoting ethical excellence and patient-centered care.

Dynamic ethical frameworks synthesize classic ethical theories and contemporary challenges in AI-driven healthcare. Healthcare organizations can develop robust frameworks that adapt to evolving ethical landscapes with agility and precision by integrating principles from consequentialism, deontology, virtue ethics, and principlism. Through iterative refinement and continuous evaluation, dynamic ethical frameworks ensure that AI-driven healthcare delivery upholds the highest standards of ethical conduct and promotes equitable outcomes for all individuals within the healthcare ecosystem.

AI-Enhanced Decision Support

Ethical decision-making lies at the heart of healthcare practice, and AI-driven decision support tools can offer invaluable assistance in navigating complex moral dilemmas. Enhanced decision support systems leverage predictive analytics and machine learning algorithms to provide real-time ethical guidance to healthcare professionals. By analyzing vast amounts of data and synthesizing relevant information, these tools empower clinicians to make evidence-based decisions rather than decisions based on hunches and experience alone, that prioritize patient well-being and uphold ethical principles. By promoting ethical excellence at the point of care, enhanced decision support systems improve patient outcomes and foster trust in the healthcare system.

Enhanced decision-making support in healthcare involves leveraging AI-driven tools to provide real-time guidance to clinicians, particularly in navigating complex ethical dilemmas. One approach that embodies this concept is the SHARE approach, advocated by the Agency for Healthcare Research and Quality. The SHARE approach—Seek, Help, Assess, Reach, and Evaluate—provides a structured framework for integrating evidence-based practices into clinical decision-making processes.

SEEKING THE PATIENT'S PARTICIPATION

The first step in the SHARE approach involves seeking relevant evidence to inform clinical decisions and the patient's participation. AI-driven decision support systems leverage machine learning algorithms to analyze vast amounts of clinical data and identify evidence-based practices relevant to a patient's condition. By aggregating and synthesizing data from EHRs, medical literature, and other sources, AI algorithms can assist clinicians in identifying the most relevant evidence to guide their decision-making process with the patient's participation.

HELPING THE PATIENT EXPLORE AND COMPARE TREATMENT OPTIONS

Once relevant evidence has been selected, the next step is to help highlight critical information for the patient to facilitate decision-making. AI-driven decision support tools can leverage natural language processing algorithms to extract relevant information from clinical notes, diagnostic reports, and other sources, presenting it clearly and concisely for clinicians to review. By highlighting essential information such as diagnostic test results, treatment options, and potential risks and benefits, AI algorithms can assist clinicians in quickly assessing the available evidence, exploring and comparing treatment options, and helping patients make informed decisions.

ASSESSING THE PATIENT'S VALUES

The third step in the SHARE approach involves assessing the patient's values and understanding their preferences. In the context of both the patient's values and preferences, appropriate evidence-based treatment options can be chosen for the patient. AI-driven decision support tools can employ machine learning algorithms to analyze the quality of evidence, assessing factors such as study design, sample size, and statistical significance. By providing clinicians with an objective assessment of the strength of the evidence, AI algorithms can help guide decision-making processes and identify areas where additional research may be needed to inform clinical practice.

REACHING A DECISION WITH THE PATIENT

Based on the analysis of the available evidence, the next step is to reach a decision with the patient and recommend actionable strategies for the best clinical decision-making and treatment. AI-driven decision support systems can generate personalized treatment recommendations based on the patient's unique clinical profile, medical history, and preferences. By leveraging predictive analytics algorithms, these tools can assess the likelihood of different treatment outcomes and recommend the most effective course of action for achieving optimal patient outcomes.

EVALUATING THE PATIENT'S
DECISION AND OUTCOMES

The final step in the SHARE approach involves evaluating the outcomes of the shared clinical decisions to inform future practice. AI-driven decision support systems can track patient outcomes over time, comparing the effectiveness of different treatment strategies and identifying areas for improvement. By analyzing real-world data on treatment outcomes, AI algorithms can help clinicians refine their decision-making processes and continuously improve the quality of care delivered to patients.

Indeed, in the example of my patient in the emergency department, the SHARE approach, if applied, may have yielded a different outcome. Of course, all the tools and mechanisms to access the vital piece of information in the form of the patient's advanced directive would need to exist. Here is where our robust technological tools can be applied. In other industries information is readily available when it comes to providing service to individuals. Yet in healthcare this is ever elusive.

Enhanced decision-making support, exemplified by the SHARE approach, aligns with the principles of the DEEDS framework by promoting ethical excellence at the point of care. By providing clinicians with real-time guidance based on evidence-based practices and patient preferences, AI-driven decision support systems empower healthcare organizations to navigate complex ethical landscapes with purpose and precision. Through the systematic selection, highlighting, analysis, recommendation, and evaluation of evidence, enhanced decision-making support enhances patient outcomes and fosters trust in the healthcare system.

By integrating the SHARE approach with the DEEDS framework, healthcare organizations can ensure that ethical considerations are prioritized in clinical decision-making processes, ultimately leading to improved patient care and outcomes.

Ethical AI Design

Ethical AI design ensures the integrity and fairness of AI-driven healthcare systems. Healthcare organizations can mitigate biases and ensure alignment with organizational values by imbuing AI systems with ethical principles. Ethical AI design encompasses transparency, accountability, and fairness, fostering trust among stakeholders and promoting equitable healthcare outcomes. By prioritizing ethical considerations throughout the development process, healthcare organizations can build AI systems that uphold the highest standards of ethical conduct and prioritize the well-being of individuals within the healthcare ecosystem.

Ethical AI design is critical to ensuring the integrity and fairness of AI-driven healthcare systems. In recent years ethicists and researchers have developed frameworks to guide the ethical design, development, and deployment of AI technologies. One such framework is the Responsible AI Framework, espoused by Dorian Peters and Karina Vold from the Institute of Electrical and Electronics Engineers, which offers a comprehensive approach to integrating ethical principles into AI design processes.

UNDERSTANDING THE RESPONSIBLE AI FRAMEWORK

The Responsible AI Framework advocates for the ethical design and deployment of AI technologies across various domains, including healthcare. The framework is based on four fundamental principles: fairness, transparency, accountability, and robustness.

Fairness is a fundamental principle of the Responsible AI Framework, emphasizing the importance of ensuring that AI systems do not produce biased or discriminatory outcomes. In healthcare, fairness is essential to promoting equitable access to healthcare services and ensuring that

AI-driven interventions benefit all patient populations equally. Ethical AI design principles such as algorithmic transparency, bias mitigation, and diversity in data collection can help ensure that AI systems uphold the principle of fairness and promote equitable healthcare outcomes.

Transparency is another core principle of the Responsible AI Framework, emphasizing the need for AI systems to be transparent and explainable in their decision-making processes. In healthcare, transparency is critical to fostering stakeholder trust and ensuring clinicians understand how AI-driven algorithms arrive at their recommendations. Ethical AI design practices such as explainable AI, model interpretability, and algorithmic transparency can help enhance transparency in AI-driven healthcare systems, empowering clinicians to make informed decisions and fostering trust in AI technologies.

Accountability is a vital principle of the Responsible AI Framework, highlighting the importance of holding AI developers and deployers accountable for the outcomes of AI systems. In healthcare, accountability is essential to ensuring that AI-driven interventions adhere to ethical standards and legal regulations. Ethical AI design practices such as algorithmic auditing, stakeholder engagement, and governance mechanisms can help ensure that AI developers and deployers are held accountable for the ethical implications of their technologies, promoting responsible AI deployment and mitigating potential harm to patients.

Robustness is the final principle of the Responsible AI Framework, emphasizing the need for AI systems to be robust and resilient to adversarial attacks and unintended consequences. In healthcare, robustness is critical to ensuring the reliability and effectiveness of AI-driven interventions in real-world clinical settings. Ethical AI design practices such as robust testing, validation, and ongoing monitoring can help enhance the robustness of AI-driven healthcare systems, minimizing the risk of errors and failures that could negatively impact patient safety and outcomes.

The Responsible AI Framework aligns closely with the principles of the DEEDS framework, emphasizing the importance of ethical considerations in AI-driven healthcare design and deployment. By incorporating principles of fairness, transparency, accountability, and robustness into AI design processes, healthcare organizations can ensure that AI systems uphold the highest standards of ethical conduct and prioritize the well-being of individuals within the healthcare ecosystem. Through ethical AI design practices, healthcare organizations can build trust among stakeholders, promote equitable healthcare outcomes, and navigate complex ethical landscapes with purpose and precision. By integrating the Responsible AI Framework with the DEEDS framework, healthcare organizations can operationalize ethics in AI-driven healthcare and promote ethical excellence in designing and deploying AI technologies.

Supporting Stakeholder Engagement

Stakeholder engagement is essential to developing and implementing ethical AI-driven healthcare systems and is an example of the power of partnerships. By leveraging AI to foster inclusive dialogue and feedback mechanisms, healthcare organizations can ensure that ethical frameworks reflect diverse perspectives and values. Stakeholder engagement initiatives facilitate transparency and collaboration, empowering communities to shape healthcare policies and practices actively. Through meaningful engagement, healthcare organizations can build trust, foster accountability, and promote shared decision-making, strengthening the ethical foundation of AI-driven healthcare delivery.

Expanding supporting stakeholder engagement is vital. Stakeholder engagement is a cornerstone of ethical AI-driven healthcare, ensuring that diverse perspectives and values are incorporated into the development and implementation of healthcare systems. One framework that underscores the importance of stakeholder engagement is the Stakeholder Engagement Framework espoused by the Patient-Centered Outcomes Research Institute (PCORI), which guides engaging stakeholders in research and decision-making processes to improve patient-centered outcomes.

The PCORI Stakeholder Engagement Framework emphasizes the importance of engaging patients, caregivers, clinicians, researchers, policymakers, and other stakeholders in all stages of the research and decision-making process. The framework is based on four key principles: inclusiveness, responsiveness, partnership, and sustainability.

A foundational principle of the PCORI Stakeholder Engagement Framework, inclusiveness emphasizes the importance of including diverse perspectives and voices in decision-making. In healthcare, inclusiveness ensures that the needs and preferences of all stakeholders, including patients, caregivers, and community members, are considered in the development and implementation of AI-driven healthcare systems. Ethical AI design practices such as community engagement, patient advisory boards, and participatory research methods can ensure stakeholders from diverse backgrounds actively shape healthcare policies and practices.

Responsiveness, another core principle of the PCORI Stakeholder Engagement Framework, highlights the importance of listening to and addressing stakeholders' needs and concerns in a timely manner. In healthcare, responsiveness ensures that stakeholders' input is taken seriously and incorporated into decision-making processes. Ethical AI design practices such as feedback mechanisms, town hall meetings, and surveys can help healthcare organizations gather input from stakeholders and respond to their feedback in a transparent and accountable manner, fostering trust and collaboration.

Partnership, a vital principle of the PCORI Stakeholder Engagement Framework, emphasizes the importance of building collaborative relationships among stakeholders based on mutual respect and trust. The partnership ensures that stakeholders work together toward common goals, such as improving patient outcomes and promoting ethical healthcare practices. Ethical AI design practices such as codesign workshops, interdisciplinary collaborations, and shared decision-making processes can foster partnerships among stakeholders, empowering them to collaborate on developing and implementing AI-driven healthcare systems.

Sustainability, the final principle of the PCORI Stakeholder Engagement Framework, highlights the importance of maintaining long-term relationships with stakeholders and ensuring that their involvement is meaningful and impactful over time. In healthcare, sustainability ensures that stakeholder engagement efforts are ongoing and integrated into organizational processes and culture. Ethical AI design practices such as stakeholder training programs, capacity-building initiatives, and ongoing communication channels can help healthcare organizations sustain stakeholder engagement efforts and ensure stakeholders remain actively involved in shaping healthcare policies and practices.

The PCORI Stakeholder Engagement Framework aligns closely with the principles of the DEEDS framework, emphasizing the importance of stakeholder engagement in promoting ethical AI-driven healthcare. By incorporating inclusiveness, responsiveness, partnership, and sustainability into stakeholder engagement efforts, healthcare organizations can ensure that diverse perspectives and values are integrated into developing and implementing AI-driven healthcare systems.

Through meaningful engagement, healthcare organizations can build trust, foster accountability, and promote shared decision-making, strengthening the ethical foundation of AI-driven healthcare delivery. By integrating the PCORI Stakeholder Engagement Framework with the DEEDS framework, healthcare organizations can operationalize ethics in AI-driven healthcare and promote ethical excellence in stakeholder engagement processes.

Training and Development Foster Ethical Decisions

Training and development are essential components of fostering a culture of ethical decision-making within healthcare organizations. By utilizing AI-driven simulations and immersive learning experiences, healthcare providers can develop the knowledge and skills needed to navigate complex ethical dilemmas with confidence and compassion. Training programs leverage virtual simulations to simulate real-world scenarios, allowing clinicians to practice ethical decision-making in a safe and supportive environment. By investing in the ongoing education and development of healthcare professionals, organizations can cultivate a culture of ethical excellence and promote the highest standards of ethical conduct in AI-driven healthcare delivery.

The potential for transformative change lies in the convergence of AI and healthcare ethics. We can operationalize ethics into healthcare with AI if we apply our knowledge and take action intentionally. By embracing *The Art of Human Care* principles of purpose, personalization, and partnerships, along with the DEEDS framework and operationalizing ethics through AI, healthcare organizations can navigate complex ethical landscapes with purpose, precision, and compassion. The fusion of technological innovation and ethical excellence heralds a future where healthcare transcends boundaries, driven by a commitment to equity, compassion, and moral integrity.

Through intentional deeds grounded in ethical principles, healthcare organizations can realize their vision of providing high-quality, patient-centered care for all individuals within the healthcare ecosystem—even beyond the walls of their institutions.

NOTES

"United States: Statement from Governor Phil Scott for Independence Day," MENA Report, 2019.

"Why AI Is Crucial to Addressing Healthcare Inequalities," CyberNews, https://cybernews.cloud/why-ai-is-crucial-to-addressing-healthcare-inequalities/.

"Ontological Examples: A Deep Dive into Existential Concepts," TechieScience, https://lambdageeks.com/ontological-examples/.

"How Can We Retrain People for the Age of AI?" TechyTool, https://techytool.com/how-can-we-retrain-people-for-the-age-of-ai/.

"AI-Driven Social Media," Jinko AI, https://docs.jinkoai.com/ai-driven-social-media.

Scott, J. D., "Comment on: 'Gastrointestinal Symptoms before and after Laparoscopic Roux-en-Y Gastric Bypass: A Longitudinal Assessment," Surgery for Obesity and Related Diseases, 2019 https://doi.org/10.1016/j.soard.2019.04.014.

"Artificial Intelligence for Enhanced Clinical Decision-Making Processes," https://aiforsocialgood.ca/blog/artificial-intelligence-as-a-powerful-tool-enhancing-clinical-decision-making-processes.

"Shared Decision-Making in Kidney Cancer," Action Kidney Cancer, https://actionkidneycancer.org/shared-decision-making-in-kidney-cancer/.

"Online Relative Risk Calculator | Calculate the Relative Risk and Risk Ratio for a Study or Experiment," OnlineCalculatorsFree, https://www.onlinecalculatorsfree.com/math/relative-risk-calculator.html.

"TRACK-TBI NET Selected as Research Network for BARDA-Sponsored Trial of Abbott TBI Aid-in-Diagnosis Trial," TBI Endpoints Development (TED) Initiative, https://tbiendpoints.ucsf.edu/news/track-tbi-net-selected-research-network-barda-sponsored-trial-abbott-tbi-aid-diagnosis-trial.

"TDDC Partners with Southeast Texas Gastroenterology Associates," TDDC, https://tddctx.com/local-news/tddc-partners-with-southeast-texas-gastroenterology-associates.

"Controversial Event in Brussels Allegedly Funded by UAE Raises Concerns over MEPs' Integrity," Brussels Watch, June 2, 2023, https://brusselswatch.org/controversial-event-in-brussels-allegedly-funded-by-uae-raises-concerns-over-meps-integrity/.

"Trusty Planet," ES Desire, April 19, 2023, https://www.services.esdesire.com/portfolio/trusty-planet.

"What Are the Limitations of Current AI Technology?" TechyTool, https://techytool.com/what-are-the-limitations-of-current-ai-technology/.

"Canada: New Strategic Framework Sets Vision for a Sport Sector for Everyone," MENA Report, 2020.

"Staff Training: Fostering Inclusivity in Nurseries," Early Years Consultant London, https://nurseryconsultancyuk.co.uk/staff-training-for-fostering-inclusivity-in-nurseries/.

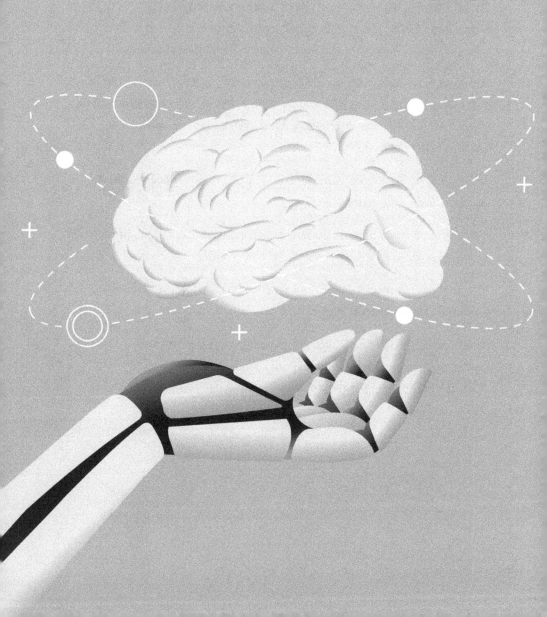

CHAPTER 8

THE VP4 FRAMEWORK: A CASE STUDY, HUMANOID ROBOTS

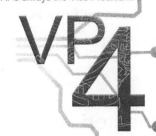

Humans are the President.
AI is always the Vice President.

Purpose

Design AI solutions with clear, ethical goals that benefit patients and align with broader health objectives.

Personalization

Leverage AI to tailor healthcare solutions to individual patient needs, improving the accuracy and relevance of treatments and interventions.

Partnership

Foster collaborative relationships between AI systems, health care professionals, and patients to enhance trust, communication, and outcomes.

Productivity

Teach AI repetitive and trainable tasks, allowing medical professionals to provide better, more personalized care to more patients.

In healthcare, the integration of AI holds immense promise for revolutionizing patient care, particularly in domains such as eldercare, where the demand for skilled labor often outstrips supply. Humanoid robots powered by AI, such as BEOMNI™ AI, represent a cutting-edge solution to address these challenges. This chapter explores a case study in which humanoid robots are deployed to augment healthcare tasks, focusing on organ transplantation procedures. By applying the VP4 conceptual framework—purpose, personalization, partnership, and productivity—we examine how these robots can uphold ethical standards, tailor care to individual needs, foster collaboration, and enhance efficiency in healthcare settings.

The VP4 framework represents a strategic paradigm shift in integrating AI into healthcare, combining human care principles with the productivity benefits of AI. Drawing an analogy from the US military's nomenclature for V fixed-wing aircraft, where "V" denotes high-flying capabilities, the VP aspect of the framework highlights AI's role as a vice president, VP to the human, an assistant that helps individuals be more productive and accomplish more. Let's delve deeper into each pillar of the VP4 framework.

Purpose: Ethical and Goal-Oriented AI

The purpose pillar emphasizes the importance of designing AI solutions with clear, ethical goals that benefit patient care and align with broader health objectives. In healthcare, AI should serve as a tool to enhance the well-being of patients and communities. This means ensuring AI applications adhere to ethical principles such as transparency, accountability, and fairness. For example, AI algorithms used for diagnosis should prioritize accuracy and patient safety while minimizing bias and discrimination. By defining a clear purpose for

AI in healthcare, stakeholders can ensure that technology serves the greater good and advances the mission of improving patient outcomes.

The deployment of humanoid robots in healthcare is driven by a clear purpose: to bridge the gap between demand and supply of skilled labor, ensuring access to quality care for all. This workforce expansion aligns with the ethical imperative of healthcare—equitable resource distribution and improved patient outcomes. BEOMNI™ AI embodies this purpose by offering a scalable solution for labor-intensive tasks across various healthcare domains.

Personalization: Tailoring Healthcare Solutions to Individual Needs

Personalization is an essential aspect of modern healthcare, and AI can play a crucial role in tailoring treatments and interventions to individual patient needs. By analyzing large datasets and leveraging machine learning algorithms, AI can identify patterns and trends that may not be apparent to human practitioners. Data and information enable healthcare providers to deliver more accurate and relevant care to each patient, leading to improved outcomes and patient satisfaction. For example, AI-powered decision support systems can help clinicians select the most effective treatment options based on a patient's unique characteristics and medical history. Personalized medicine, empowered by AI, has the potential to revolutionize healthcare by delivering targeted interventions that maximize efficacy and minimize side effects.

Humanoid robots equipped with BEOMNI™ AI demonstrate the capacity to personalize healthcare interventions. In the context of organ transplantation, these robots adapt to individual patient needs by learning and mastering specific tasks over time. They enhance surgical precision and efficiency by leveraging haptic feedback and object recognition. Furthermore, their ability to learn by observation accelerates skill acquisition, ensuring a customized approach to patient care.

Partnership: Collaborative Relationships between Humans and AI

The partnership pillar emphasizes fostering collaborative relationships among AI systems, healthcare professionals, and patients. AI should not replace human caregivers but rather complement their skills and expertise. By working together synergistically, humans and AI can achieve better outcomes than either could alone. For example, AI-powered virtual assistants can help patients manage chronic conditions by providing personalized reminders, medication schedules, and lifestyle recommendations. Similarly, AI can assist healthcare providers by analyzing medical imaging scans, detecting abnormalities, and generating diagnostic reports. By fostering trust, communication, and mutual respect between humans and AI, we can harness the full potential of technology to improve healthcare delivery and patient outcomes.

Integrating humanoid robots fosters collaborative relationships among AI systems, healthcare professionals, and patients. These robots function as invaluable assistants in the operating room, navigating complex environments, ensuring safety protocols, and seamlessly supporting surgical teams. Through continuous learning and adaptation, they become trusted partners in delivering care, augmenting human capabilities without compromising patient safety or comfort.

Productivity: Enhancing Efficiency and Effectiveness

The productivity pillar highlights how applying the VP4 conceptual framework and leveraging AI can increase productivity across many healthcare tasks. AI has the potential to automate routine administrative tasks, streamline clinical workflows, and optimize resource allocation, allowing healthcare providers to focus more time and attention on patient care. For example, AI-powered predictive analytics can help hospitals forecast patient volumes, optimize staffing levels, and allocate resources more efficiently. Similarly, AI-driven decision support systems can assist clinicians in diagnosing and treating patients more quickly and accurately, reducing wait times and improving overall throughput. By enhancing efficiency and effectiveness, AI can help healthcare organizations deliver higher-quality care at a lower cost, ultimately improving patient outcomes and satisfaction.

A key advantage of humanoid robots powered by BEOMNI™ AI lies in their ability to improve productivity in healthcare settings. Automating routine tasks such as inventory management and instrument sterilization frees up human resources for more complex and human-centric aspects of care delivery. Moreover, their multitasking abilities and scalability enable them to handle diverse responsibilities simultaneously, optimizing workflow efficiency and resource utilization.

The VP4 framework provides a comprehensive approach to integrating AI into healthcare, emphasizing the importance of purpose-driven, personalized, and collaborative AI solutions that enhance productivity and improve patient care. By leveraging AI as a strategic assistant to human caregivers, we can unlock the full potential of technology to transform healthcare delivery and improve the lives of patients around the world.

Humanoid Robots in Organ Transplantation

Our innovative work in pioneering Specialized Thoracic Adapted Recovery (STAR) Teams has significantly advanced thoracic organ transplantation. Over fifteen years, we focused on creating a regionalized heart and lung transplant service, culminating in the publication of our groundbreaking results in 2023. The methods our team employed involved the meticulous review of data on organ procurements conducted by the STAR Teams from November 2, 2004, to June 30, 2020. The results of our efforts were significant.

STAR Teams successfully recovered thoracic organs from 1,118 donors. The recovered organs included 978 hearts, 823 bilateral lungs, 89 right lungs, 92 left lungs, and 8 heart and lung combinations. Impressively, 79 percent of hearts and 76.1 percent of lungs recovered by STAR Teams were successfully transplanted, underscoring the effectiveness of their approach. The meticulous care and attention to detail exhibited by STAR Teams were evident in their remarkable twenty-four-hour graft survival rates, with lungs achieving a perfect 100 percent survival rate and hearts achieving an impressive 99 percent survival rate. The impact of our work extended far and wide, with 47 transplant centers receiving at least 1 heart and 37 centers receiving at least 1 lung procured by STAR Teams during the study period.

Our pioneering efforts in establishing STAR teams have significantly improved transplantation rates. This success underscores the importance of specialized expertise and regional collaboration in optimizing organ procurement and transplantation processes, ultimately enhancing patient outcomes and saving lives. Based on that foundational work, new opportunities are emerging, and there is potential to combine lessons learned from the past and apply this era's latest technology, AI, and data to improve transplantation even more.

In the context of organ transplantation, humanoid robots equipped with BEOMNI™ AI demonstrate advanced sensing capabilities. They navigate the operating room environment with precision, responding to haptic feedback and recognizing the required surgical tools. By adapting to the surgical setting, these robots ensure seamless integration into existing workflows, enhancing surgical efficiency and patient safety.

Humanoid robots learn and adapt to their roles in organ transplantation through observation and task repetition. By leveraging virtual reality simulations and human demonstrations, they acquire essential skills and refine their performance over time. This iterative learning process enables them to function autonomously in the operating room, supporting surgical teams consistently across diverse cases and scenarios.

BEOMNI™ AI-powered humanoid robots optimize surgical workflow through effective planning and scheduling. They assist in task prioritization, inventory management, and resource allocation, ensuring that surgical supplies are readily available for transplantation procedures. These robots can streamline the surgical process by automating routine tasks, such as instrument sterilization and restocking, minimizing delays and enhancing overall productivity.

One of the critical advantages of humanoid robots in organ transplantation is their scalability and multitasking capabilities. They can adapt to varying case volumes and surgical complexities, providing continuous support to surgical teams without interruption. Moreover, these robots can perform multiple tasks simultaneously by incorporating additional arms or functionalities, further enhancing workflow efficiency and surgical outcomes.

Integrating humanoid robots powered by BEOMNI™ AI represents a transformative example and approach to healthcare delivery, particularly in domains such as organ transplantation. By applying the VP4 conceptual framework—purpose, personalization, partnership, and productivity—we can ensure that these robots uphold ethical standards, tailor care to individual needs, foster collaboration, and enhance efficiency in healthcare settings. As we continue to innovate and refine AI technologies, humanoid robots will play an increasingly vital role in augmenting human capabilities and improving patient outcomes in healthcare, eldercare, and beyond.

Academic Partnership for Innovation

The ability to collaborate with academia cannot be understated as an integral aspect of serving as a catalyst to this transformative journey and making a lasting impact in the field of transplant medicine.

I shared some of Dr. Amol Ahmed Joshi's insights in chapter 4. He also provides a valuable framework for how academia can potentially partner with new AI innovations in healthcare. Dr. Joshi's expertise in healthcare innovation, AI, and biomedical informatics enriches the discussion on the potential applications of technologies within the healthcare landscape.

Amol emphasizes the importance of academia in driving innovation in healthcare by providing an environment for testing innovation in real-world settings. Academic institutions such as Wake Forest University with an academic medical center and community are crucial in researching, developing, and testing new technologies, including AI-driven solutions. By leveraging academia's expertise, AI innovations can benefit from cutting-edge research and collaborate with academic researchers to enhance its capabilities further.

One novel application, AI-Enabled Robotic-Assisted Cadaveric Organ Visualization and Recovery (AI-RACOVER), provides an example of the academic-AI innovation partnership in action. Imagine the potential for AI-RACOVER to contribute to the workflow of assisting in surgical organ recovery. Through partnerships with academic institutions, AI-RACOVER can access vast repositories of EHRs and relevant data on healthy organs as a training data set. By analyzing this data, AI algorithms can be developed, assisted by computer vision, to identify patterns indicative of donor organ quality and suitability for transplantation. The collaboration between an AI-RACOVER innovation and academia enables the development and validation of these AI-driven diagnostic and assessment tools, leading to improved patient outcomes.

Amol underscores the importance of standardization and experimentation in AI-driven healthcare innovations. Academic partnerships facilitate the development of standardized frameworks and toolkits for AI applications, enabling widespread adoption and experimentation. Through collaborative research initiatives, such as the AI-RACOVER example, new AI technologies could be piloted on a small scale, allowing for iterative improvements and validation before large-scale implementation and patient application. This approach minimizes risks and maximizes the impact of innovations in real-world healthcare settings.

Another area Amol identified is optimizing back-office processes using AI technology. Revenue cycle management, medical coding, and administrative tasks are ripe for AI-driven automation and efficiency improvements. By partnering with academia, commercial medical technology entities can explore innovative solutions to streamline these processes, reducing administrative burden and improving overall healthcare system performance. Academic collaboration provides access to diverse expertise and resources necessary to effectively develop and implement AI-powered back-office solutions.

Amol emphasizes the importance of ethical AI development and knowledge sharing within academia and the healthcare industry. Academic partnerships ensure innovations adhere to ethical standards and promote transparency, fairness, and patient privacy. Additionally, academia serves as a platform for sharing research findings, best practices, and lessons learned, fostering collaboration and driving continuous improvement in AI-enabled healthcare.

Leveraging partnerships with academia enhances the ability to drive novel innovation, advance research, and improve patient care within the healthcare domain. By collaborating with academic institutions, innovators can harness the collective expertise, resources, and collaborative spirit of academia to accelerate the development and implementation of AI-driven solutions for healthcare challenges.

Transforming Transplant Surgery

By applying the VP4 conceptual framework—purpose, personalization, partnership, and productivity—we can examine how the robot highlighted in the AI-RACOVER example upholds ethical standards, tailors care to individual needs, fosters collaboration, and enhances efficiency in healthcare settings.

The VP4 framework represents a strategic paradigm shift in integrating AI into healthcare, combining human care principles with the productivity benefits of AI. Thus, an AI-RACOVER application that improves the assessment of donor organs and assists surgeons with organ recovery is uniquely positioned to transform the transplant surgery landscape. Building upon an existing robotic platform, expertise, and decades of experience, we could augment a transplant surgeons' capabilities, thereby increasing the rate of viable cadaveric organ recoveries and successful transplantations. This initiative outlined below leverages the precision and efficiency of how a robotic system integrated with cutting-edge AI could improve outcomes across all organ types and patient demographics.

OBJECTIVES

1. Maximize the Utility of Existing Robotic Platforms: AI-driven decision-making tools improve precision in organ recovery.

2. Elevate Transplant Success Rates: Assist surgeons in complex procedures, increasing the viability and compatibility of transplanted organs.

3. Democratize Access to Transplant Surgery: Use data analytics to ensure fair and equitable organ allocation across diverse populations.

STRATEGY

1. AI Integration: Develop AI modules that seamlessly integrate with existing robotic platforms, focusing on data analysis, surgical planning, and real-time assistance.

2. Robotic System Enhancement: Upgrade the robotic platform to accommodate new AI features, improving adaptability to various transplant scenarios.

3. Surgeon Training Program: Create a comprehensive training curriculum for surgeons to effectively use the AI-augmented robotic system in their respective workflows.

IMPLEMENTATION PLAN

1. Phase 1—AI Development and Integration: Develop AI tools tailored to the robotic platform. Includes machine learning models for patient data analysis and surgical strategy optimization.

2. Phase 2—Pilot Implementation: Partner with select transplant centers within an academic setting to integrate the enhanced system into real-world surgeries and collect extensive feedback for system refinement.

3. Phase 3—Expansion and Scale-Up: Gradually introduce the system across a broader range of medical centers, accompanied by thorough training and support services.

In this example an AI-RACOVER application may be poised to revolutionize transplant surgery by increasing the rate of viable cadaveric organ recoveries and successful transplantations, bridging a critical gap in healthcare.

NOTES

Tetteh H.A., Brandenhoff P., and Higgins R.S., "Specialized Thoracic Adapted Recovery Model for Thoracic Organ Recovery: A 15-Year Review," Transplantation Processes 55, no. 2 (March 2023): 384–386. doi: 10.1016/j. transproceed.2023.02.011.

Kaboudan, A., & Eldin, W. S., "AI-Driven Medical Imaging Platform: Advancements in Image Analysis and Healthcare Diagnosis, *Journal of the ACS Advances in Computer Science* 1, no.14 (2023), https://doi. org/10.21608/asc.2024.248278.1018.

"Importance of Pharmacy in Daily Life," Study Medicine in Europe, https:// www.studying-medicine.com/importance-of-pharmacy-in-daily-life/.

"The Benefits of Using AI in Land-Based Aquaculture?" Agri Expo, https:// trends.agriexpo.online/project-68380.html.

"Can AI Revolutionize the Way We Work?" S&B Finishing, https://www. powdercoatchicago.com/can-ai-revolutionize-the-way-we-work/.

"The Impact of Generative AI on Content Creation: Revolutionizing the Creative Landscape," https://www.explainx.ai/post/the-impact-of-generative-ai-on-content-creation-revolutionizing-the-creative-landscape.

Harsh Majethiya, "Data Cloud & Generative AI Services," Healthcare IT Leaders, https://www.healthcareitleaders.com/practice-areas/data-cloud-generative-ai-consulting/.

"Say Goodbye to Medical Note-Taking: Try Virtual Medical Scribe," Scribe Align, https://scribealign.com/virtual-medical-scribe.

"Gene Snyder: Discovering the Legacy of a Prominent Figure," December 20, 2023, https://scienceofbiogenetics.com/articles/meet-gene-snyder-a-pioneer-and-innovator-in-the-world-of-technology-and-entrepreneurship.

"During the Industrial Revolution the Demand for Skilled Labor," Android62, January 20, 2024, https://android62.com/en/question/during-the-industrial-revolution-the-demand-for-skilled-labor/.

"How Resource Management Is Revolutionized in the Internet of Things," Insight Tribune, June 18, 2023, https://www.nalug.net/how-resource-management-is-revolutionized-in-the-internet-of-things/.

"Perks of White-Glove Furniture Delivery," Domestic Distribution, https://domesticdistribution.co.uk/luxury-at-your-doorstep-unleashing-the-magic-of-white-glove-furniture-delivery/.

"Amazon's Digit Pilot: A Landmark Experiment for Humanoid Robots," BEST Webhosting, October 22, 2023, https://best-webhosting.org/technology/amazons-digit-pilot-a-landmark-experiment-for-humanoid-robots/.

"Harnessing AI for Enhanced Weather Predictions," ThinkML, February 2, 2024, https://thinkml.ai/harnessing-ais-power-transforming-historic-weather-data-into-predictive-insights/.

"Reviving Failed IT Projects: Harnessing the Power of Dynamics 365 Project Rescue," February 9, 2024 Dynamics in Motion, https://www.dim.ltd/reviving-failed-it-projects-harnessing-the-power-of-dynamics-365-project-rescue/.

"EGOS—Submission of Full Papers," European Group for Organizational Studies, https://www.egos.org/jart/prj3/egos/main.jart?rel=de&reserve-mode=active&content-id=1581807636344&subtheme_id=1542700474982.

"Who Are the Best Leaders from Life Sciences in India 2023?" New York Times Now, https://www.newyorktimesnow.com/who-are-the-best-leaders-from-life-sciences-in-india-2023/.

CHAPTER 9

THE VP4 FRAMEWORK: TRANSFORMATIVE INNOVATION IN HEALTHCARE

In the rapidly evolving healthcare landscape, innovation is not merely a buzzword. It's a necessity. With the advent of advanced technologies such as AI, the potential for transformative change in healthcare delivery has never been more significant. This chapter explores how two pioneering companies, Layer Health and Authenticx, are reshaping the healthcare ecosystem through platform innovation and the greater utility of AI.

In healthcare, where empathy is as essential as medical expertise, the challenge of providing empathy at scale has long perplexed industry leaders. However, with the advent of innovative AI solutions such as Authenticx, pioneered by Amy Brown, a new paradigm is emerging. Authenticx uses AI and natural language processing to analyze millions of recorded customer interactions—calls, emails, or chats—

and discern insights and meaningful information. By harnessing the VP4 conceptual framework—purpose, personalization, partnership, and productivity—Authenticx exemplifies how listening at scale can lead to empathy at scale.

Purpose drives meaningful impact. Amy Brown's journey to founding Authenticx is a testament to that power of purpose. Born out of her twenty years of experience within the healthcare system, Authenticx embodies Brown's commitment to addressing the administrative waste and missed opportunities plaguing healthcare delivery. Her background in macro social work and extensive tenure in healthcare operations gave her a unique vantage point in identifying systemic inefficiencies.

Amy's unique perspective comes from leading call centers, which are often the front door to healthcare for many patients. She is a prime example of leveraging AI to deliver better healthcare and empower patients. I had the opportunity to speak with Amy when she appeared as a guest on my Forbes Books *Smarter Healthcare with AI* podcast. Here's what she had to say:

> Authenticx is an expression of my response to twenty years of working in the healthcare system. I started as the daughter of a physician who helped to bring me along and see, from his perspective, what patient care looked like firsthand for patients. I decided not to pursue a clinical career and ended up getting my education in macro social work.
>
> I really cared about systems of care and started my career in state government, working on Medicaid policy with underserved populations. I then jumped into the private sector and worked with Medicare, Medicaid, and commercial

health plans in operations roles. Over twenty years of doing that work, I came to see a few things.

I saw firsthand the administrative waste that our health system has developed over the years. I saw a lot of missed opportunities to connect the clinical side of healthcare with what's going on in the administrative side. In my roles as a call center leader, I realized that the story of the breakdown in patient care could be told through the millions of customer conversations that were being transacted and facilitated by the healthcare enterprise.

So I left my career when I was forty-two years old, a mom of four kids, my husband a stay-at-home dad. I said, "I'm not going to die happy if I don't try to solve this problem or at least make a dent in it." That's the backstory behind Authenticx.

Authenticx views recorded customer conversation data as a lost source of insight that the healthcare system desperately needs to listen to. There's a lot of patient experience, effort, and resources being spent on surveying patients and customers, on building customer journeys, but if we're not leveraging the literal customer voices that are flowing into our billing lines, our customer service, our scheduling, our nurse triage lines, if we're not leveraging those recorded conversations, then we're missing a really important and rich source of insight.

Authenticx works with care companies—hospital and health systems, health insurers, and pharmaceutical companies—to take their conversation data into our platform. We use AI as ears that can listen to 100 percent of customer conversations and then digest and succinctly tell the story back to the health companies we work with about what is going on in these customer conversations that is causing friction, is causing patients to lapse in therapy or care, or to drop out of the care plan. It's really about connecting that administrative side of the business with the clinical care side of the business.

Historically, healthcare organizations think of administrative customer service as separate and distinct from clinical care.

What we know from listening—and we listened to 250 million customer conversations last year—in those administrative conversations, customers, patients, and caregivers are telling their story about the clinical experience, about how difficult it is to navigate care, and why they're dropping out of care or can't get access to care.

We've made so much of a big deal in this country about the impact of social determinants of health. We've got to look at ourselves in the mirror and ask, "How are we contributing to the gaps in care by our own processes and systems?"

That's what we're trying to shine a light on and solve. Those problems are solvable if we listen to the data that's right under our noses.

From those 250 million conversations, at a high level, we have learned that the system itself is crushingly complex for the consumers to navigate. When you distill it down to individual organizations or individual lines of business where organizations have organized workforces to help serve a particular purpose in the customer journey, our clients are able to use our platform to define the root cause drivers of patient friction. What is driving patients to disenroll from our program? For them to say, "Hey, I'm not going to go to my follow-up visits," or "Hey, I'm not going to fill this prescription, even though my doctor prescribed it."

We're getting to the root reasons for those, quantifying the issues at scale. Now we have a universe of data that is no longer anecdotal, that is no longer a fraction of customers that are responding to surveys. We have the universe of data where we can quantify what pain points are driving the biggest volume of issues.

We can even tie that to dollars spent by the health system in trying to resolve those issues. What we're seeing leaders do is take this data to inform their action plans and strategy to unstick their patient journey. We're seeing those clients who are listening reduce their call volume on pain-point issues and redeploy their nurses to actually answering nurse-level questions versus administrative questions.

One of my favorite stories is of a nurse triage line that a hospital system had set up to help answer questions in between clinical visits. We were listening at scale to 100 percent of them. One of the cool things when you're listening on an ongoing basis is you can see when topics or issues are trending up at a macro view.

With one health system, our platform noticed a rise in the number of distressed callers around the access to mental healthcare. When diving into that subset of conversations, we could see that these were parents who were calling on behalf of their children, during and right after the COVID crisis, who were desperately in need of mental healthcare.

As the calls were coming in, the nurses were trying to respond. But what really needed to happen was that the next layer up of leadership needed to understand the quantity and the severity of the curve in terms of the need. Once they realized that, they were able to wrap their arms around a more systemic response to that patient population. They were able to organize a coalition of providers internally and respond more effectively. It allowed the system to innovate.

I learned this is really exposing information. It's their own data. It's not like I'm getting it from some other source. It is hard and takes really strong cultures within these systems to be able to receive this challenging information. So I've learned how to prepare clients for what they're going to hear.

There are always really positive stories that would otherwise never be heard too. In that moment there's a very human exchange where a patient is being helped. What we've seen happen with organizations who use listening at scale as a tactic and a strategy, they're using those good stories to inspire their entire workforce. Whether you're in auditing, back office, front office, or you're a clinician, everybody gets out of bed because they want to help someone. You can use these voices and these stories to help inspire an entire culture—and we're seeing organizations do that.

We created a feature called the call montage feature. And what it does, it looks at all the conversations and finds the segments of the conversations that have been tagged or labeled with that frustrating comment or complaint. They're able to be compiled like an old-school mixtape or like your Spotify playlist.

A leader can go in and say, "I want to hear what yesterday's complaints sounded like." Instead of hunting through a telephony platform, they can see the graph that tells them that about 20 percent of yesterday's customers were complaining. Now they can click through their montage library and listen to samples of what that really sounds like.

We found that the marriage of visualized, quantified data with the literal patient voice is what is driving people to act within their organizations. There's something human about connecting if you're a C-suite, and you hardly ever touch or feel or get around your patients.

When you can connect with them, it makes you want to act. The data comes to life in the human form, and you can't unhear it.

Productivity can be viewed as amplifying human potential. While the VP4 framework underscores the centrality of human-centric principles, it also acknowledges technology's transformative potential. Authenticx epitomizes this synergy by harnessing AI to augment human capabilities rather than supplant them. By automating the labor-intensive task of analyzing customer conversations, Authenticx liberates healthcare professionals to focus on higher-order activities that demand human ingenuity and empathy.

As Amy Brown's journey exemplifies, the quest for empathy at scale is not merely a technological endeavor but a profoundly human one. By listening attentively to the voices of patients and caregivers, Authenticx illuminates the path toward a more compassionate and responsive healthcare system. Authenticx heralds a future where empathy is a virtue and a fundamental imperative in healthcare delivery through purpose-driven innovation, personalized insights, collaborative partnerships, and productivity enhancements.

Layer Health: Unlocking the Potential of Unstructured Medical Data

David Sontag, a trailblazing figure at the intersection of AI and healthcare, is the cofounder and CEO of Layer Health. He spearheads a groundbreaking initiative to leverage AI to unlock the potential of unstructured medical data. David's extensive expertise extends beyond his leadership role—he holds a distinguished position at MIT, where he has authored more than one hundred influential publications in AI and machine learning.

David and I met during a summit before the pandemic that convened intellectuals, academics, technologists, and AI experts to discuss how we could digitize the immense repository of data in the JPC for the greater good. I had the opportunity to talk with David again in early 2024 when he was my guest on the Forbes Books *Smarter Healthcare with AI* podcast that I host. I asked what has changed with respect to AI and healthcare postpandemic. Here's what David had to say:

It's been quite a journey in the AI field over the past few years, both as an academic and an entrepreneur. The technology has evolved substantially. Our company is built on large language models, which didn't exist five years ago and have completely revolutionized the way we tackle problems involving language and vision.

Moreover, I'd say the entire field has changed in the healthcare field. The willingness and appetite to bring AI into the clinic is unprecedented. Healthcare organizations in the US, both private and public, have transformed and made it possible to actually start thinking about how we integrate AI at scale, actually changing the point of care and beyond.

I first started getting into AI back in the late '90s, early 2000s, when I was a high school student and then a college student at Rutgers and UC Berkeley. I was really excited about how AI brings together both really cool applications but also some very deep mathematics.

The first couple of use cases I focused on were in the financial domain and then in web search through internships at Google. I continued diving deep into AI, doing AI research when I was an undergraduate at UC Berkeley.

The AI that I was thinking about at the time was how do we build computers that can reason like humans reason, recognizing that we were incredibly good at making inferences and doing options. Computers typically are not very good at that.

When I started my career and transitioned to becoming a faculty member at NYU, I was looking to have one foot in an application with real deep social impact and the other foot in the more theoretical side of AI, where we could push the boundaries of AI techniques. That's when I landed in AI and healthcare.

I was fortunate at MIT to have incredible collaborations with health systems and health insurers. With that came access to data and clarity around the problems, which, if we could solve, would have a big impact on healthcare. The translation of those into clinical practices went beyond the small number of health systems and insurers that I worked with. So my research then looked at what could we do on the AI side that would actually accelerate that translation.

At my company, Layer Health, we're tackling this problem of very deeply understanding what's going on with patients—what's happened to them in the past, what's going on with them now, and what's going to happen to them in the future—by building a layer of high quality, validated information about patients that all other aspects of medicine and healthcare can build on top of.

We first started tackling this problem in 2012, when I was working very closely with one of my cofounders, Stephen Horn, a physician at Beth Israel Deaconess Medical Center. He's trained as a computer scientist, did a clinical informatics fellowship, and practices in emergency medicine at that hospital.

We started thinking about how we could bring AI into the emergency department, where there were a number of challenges. The clinical community would come to us saying, "OK, you do machine learning. These problems look like they are just right for machine learning—help us with diagnosis and risk stratification."

As an early example, we worked on early detection of sepsis, which today is a very commonly discussed application of machine learning in healthcare. As we tackled these early use cases of machine learning, we realized that the impact was going to be relatively small because machine learning from a predictive perspective only provides a small improvement over what you could have done with well-known clinical decision support rules that the clinical community had been developing for a long time.

What was much, much more important was how do you get instruments into the clinical workflow at the right time and what do you do with the predictions. We realized that getting the right information at the right time would be transformative.

The hospital system had a large number of decision pathways. For example, a cellulitis pathway, if a patient is suspected of having cellulitis; a cardiac pathway for patients who have cardiac etiologies; or identifying patients who are at fall risk, so when they're being transported from place to place, to use fall precautions.

For each one of these pathways, there are well-established best practices that, if you know the patient, fit into those categories. But none of those elements were recorded in structured data anywhere in the electronic medical record. There was no way to trigger decision support at the right time or in the right part of the workflow. We realized that if we could predict clinical state variables and summarize those elements with high accuracy at the point of care, we could build the next generation of electronic medical records on top of that information. That's what we set out to do.

Next, we started to rethink documentation and how we do precharting and bring the right information to clinicians' fingertips for other downstream use cases.

Machine learning really depends on having a notion of ground truth. If you don't have a good ground truth, then you can't get started. Typically, for each one of these use cases, one needs to hire a large number of research assistants at your health system or hospital to get ground truth and build machine learning models. Then, when you want to translate that to a new health system, you need to start from scratch. That was the real core issue around scalability, which our research and then later Layer Health has been transforming.

How do you scale these things? We're focused on clinical notes or unstructured clinical data. The way we get around it is by not doing labeling at all—completely skipping that process. We can do that with large language models because we have the opportunity now to have someone come in, a clinical expert. We abstract specific information about a patient, not just one patient, but maybe thousands or hundreds of thousands of patients. Our models now are good enough that we can take that English language description, couple it with the language written in the clinical notes for all of those hundreds or hundreds of thousands of patients, and immediately get the right results, get to the abstraction because we understand language so well.

We no longer need to do that huge amount of work up front to label a ton of data or to teach machine learning models to do that.

There is no one-size-fits-all solution for healthcare. Every need is distinctive. First, we're enabling our users within health systems to very quickly validate for themselves that the results are what they expect them to be without having to do a very expensive and manual validation process.

Once you recognize you need to do chart review for a particular data element from a particular predefined population, our platform is making it fast for you to quickly review the results across a large number of patients and to recognize whether the results are what you expected them to be.

How do you monitor it over time? If we can enable our customers to do that themselves, then we can start to remove one of the bottlenecks in scalability, which is expecting that the vendor is going to always have what they need for their particular use case. This we think is going to allow for an enormous amount of scalability in the healthcare system.

Regulation and FDA approval is going to be a really interesting space to watch in AI and healthcare. Starting to look at the processes by which one builds the models, validates the models, and then monitors the models is going to be where we're going to end up sitting.

If we're building the right process, we can validate that process and make sure that it leads to high-quality data and patient outcomes, which gets you the validation component and scalability.

Most importantly, the validation that is happening at one health system is going to impact other health systems. So we're creating a network effect that we think is going to lift up healthcare for everyone in the US.

Three Buckets: Quality Improvement, Site of Care Optimization, and Standardization

There are three buckets of use cases where we are going to see short-term ROI in our healthcare. The first one is on quality improvement. We're working with a health system in Wisconsin, Froedtert, associated with the Medical College of Wisconsin, doing chart abstraction for a surgical registry.

Surgery is expensive and also critical in terms of patient outcomes. One can justify the large expense that it takes to actually start to gather that data, which is essential to the quality improvement efforts. Collecting this data typically requires a huge amount of chart review. You have an army of folks to get all this information. They're pouring over the patient's medical records to abstract hundreds of different data elements that summarize the indications for surgery, other comorbidities that the patient might have, and what happened during surgery.

If you're comparing different hospitals, you better compare apples to apples. So you need that army of individuals to help do that chart abstraction. That's the part that is not scalable in healthcare. It costs a lot of money. The very high qualified nurses who would be doing that work are the same people in short demand in the US healthcare system where we have a huge nursing shortage. So how do we both scale that up within surgery and in other clinical areas where these same quality improvement efforts could be transformational to healthcare? How do we get the most important information? Structured data that you can collect cheaply and easily is not necessarily measuring what really matters.

Imagine if you had the ability to do scalable chart review cheaply and very accurately using AI. How could you rethink the next generation of registries? What could new quality improvement look like? That's what we're doing on this front.

Bucket number two is site of care optimization—providing patients the right care at the right place at the right time. Think about ambulatory surgical centers, which are outside of the hospital environment and, when suitable, much better for patients. Better patient experience can lead to better outcomes. Maybe the risk of infection is lower. If you can get surgeries that don't need the complexity of the main hospital environment outside of the hospital, you will suddenly have a lot more beds for surgeries that are much more complex.

To determine which patients are suited to an ambulatory surgical care center, you have to know their health history. Do they have a difficult airway, previous problems with anesthesia, kidney disease? These types of things may not be the best suited for ambulatory care. If we could reliably do chart review to answer each of those questions—and there's a much larger database thanks to AI—then we could get the information to the person making the decision about where this surgery should be scheduled.

Another example is hospital at-home programs. As a health system becomes more mature and increases their capabilities and technology, they can help patients stay at home. With current capabilities, this is very challenging.

But there's a will among people, academics, among industry, among health systems, among government, and among patients. The fact that there's a will now to actually do it means that we can start to dream about, as a society, not what healthcare is like today but what it could be like tomorrow.

The third bucket, AI can improve patient care and healthcare operations by fortifying standardization. Standardization provides guidelines for everything from cancer care, administration, and antibiotics to diabetic care and managing heart failure. Standardization is clinical studies and physician groups coming together to discuss best practices.

The challenge is that we're often not following these best practices. If we could quickly identify patients who are not following the current best practices, then it would provide an opportunity for standardizing care, both at the population health level and at the point of care.

Safety necessitates validation, validation that goes end to end looking at patient outcomes as impacted by AI in the loop, looking at AI and the workflow of the clinician who's using it. How do we get AI into the hands of everyone who can really benefit from AI from the healthcare perspective?

AI Augmenting Patients Directly

We also have to go well beyond thinking about AI as being integrated into the healthcare delivery system and start thinking about AI as directly augmenting patients themselves. I've been excited for a long time about the idea of patients having access to their electronic medical records. This can help patients better understand what's going on with their health in a way that helps them become much more proactive and helps them identify what resources would improve their care. This is going to lead to more equitable healthcare in the US.

Today, only those of us who have friends and family who are physicians, live in an academic environment, or have the money to pay for the right resources have a leg up, and that's not fair. How can we start to even that playing field? Information is going to be a big part of that.

One of the studies that we've been doing recently at MIT is looking at how we can take the clinical notes that physicians are writing and help patients better understand them.

Say you are a patient recently diagnosed with breast cancer. You go to meet with your oncologist for the first time. You come home and wonder, "What the heck just happened? What was my diagnosis? What's my prognosis? What am I supposed to follow up with next? What were my options and why were those my options?"

Often patients come to health visits with a family member or some other caregiver who can help them with documenting information during the visit, but not everyone has that benefit.

We recently did a study using a large language model, GPT-4 for OpenAI, within a patient-facing application to help patients better understand their notes along four axes. One, helped translate the note into consumer vocabulary. Two, it defined certain terms, clarifying words that might be quite technical. Three, it automatically generated questions and answers—questions that you might have after reading this note. Four, it provides a bulleted list of follow-ups, what you are supposed to do next after the visit.

We used large language models to develop all four of these. Then we did a study, first with two hundred healthy women who did not have breast cancer but who were representative of the population who might be newly diagnosed with breast cancer. We used de-identified clinical notes donated by previous breast cancer survivors and some synthetically created clinical notes.

First, we showed them the notes. Then we showed them the notes that had been augmented by GPT-4 for OpenAI to provide the four interventions. Next, we asked a number of follow-up questions to simulate how well they understood the notes in terms of how they would impact various decisions that they would have to make in the near future had they been newly diagnosed with breast cancer.

We found a significant improvement in the women using the notes augmented by the large language models versus those not using it.

Second, we took the same steps with a small number of women who had breast cancer. We interviewed them. We had oncologists who listened to each of these phone calls to ensure that the AI we were using was not presenting incorrect information.

We interviewed them. First, we showed them their original notes and asked them to tell us about the questions they had during that visit and what they did. They shared their questions about their diagnosis and all the Googling they did to try to understand their next steps.

Next, they clicked a button on the platform that showed them the automatically generated questions, answers, and follow-up items. You could see these patients' eyes light up. One woman said that she had never understood her diagnosis until that moment.

Another woman said that this would have substantially reduced the stress of the moment because it helped introduce the information in a much more calming way instead of

Googling around to sites where she didn't know whether the information was relevant to her case.

Another patient mentioned that it raised new questions about whether the AI was correct and that new stressors might be involved if the AI were to bring up information that they hadn't considered before.

Using AI like this could be hugely impactful from an equity perspective, really improving healthcare for everyone, everywhere. It's an example of what it means for AI safety and development, and I'd like to see both academics and companies working in this space start to replicate it.

What gives me optimism and hope for the future of AI and healthcare is that there's a will among academics, industry, health systems, government, and patients to take these wonderful advances that we've had in technology in recent years and experiment in ways that might be a little bit scary because they do challenge the status quo. They do need to be done carefully, thoughtfully, and safely. But the fact that there's a will to actually do it means that we can start to dream as a society—not about what healthcare is like today but what it could be like tomorrow.

Synergies and Opportunities: The Power of Collaboration

While Layer Health and Authenticx may approach healthcare innovation from different angles, their shared commitment to leveraging AI to drive positive change creates numerous opportunities for collaboration and synergy. By combining Layer Health's expertise in unlocking insights from medical data with Authenticx's focus on amplifying the patient voice, healthcare organizations can better understand the factors influencing patient outcomes and experiences, as well as gain deeper insights into the effectiveness of clinical interventions, identify areas for improvement, and tailor care delivery strategies to meet patients' needs better. Likewise, by leveraging Authenticx's patient feedback data to inform the development of AI algorithms, Layer Health can enhance the accuracy and relevance of its predictive models, ultimately leading to more personalized and effective healthcare solutions.

By collaborating with researchers, policymakers, technology partners, and other stakeholders in the healthcare ecosystem, Layer Health and Authenticx can drive collective action to address some of the most pressing challenges facing healthcare today, from improving access to care and reducing disparities in health outcomes to enhancing the quality and safety of healthcare delivery. The possibilities for collaboration and innovation are endless.

Layer Health and Authenticx exemplify the transformative potential of AI-driven innovation in healthcare. Through their respective platform innovations, these companies are revolutionizing how healthcare data is analyzed and interpreted. They are also humanizing healthcare by amplifying the patient voice and empowering healthcare organizations to deliver more personalized, patient-centered care. By embracing collaboration and synergy, Layer Health and Authenticx are paving the way for a brighter, more equitable future for healthcare.

NOTES

"How ISO 22000:2018 Addresses Food Safety Concerns," ISO Consultant in UAE Dubai Abu Dhabi ISO 9001 14001 45001 HACCP, https://iso-uae-dubai.com/how-iso-220002018-addresses-food-safety-concerns/.

"Negative Feedback and Brand Image Repair," Local SEO and Marketing | Blue Ocean HQ, https://blueoceanhq.com/negative-feedback-and-brand-image-repair/.

"Tina White and the Importance of Consulting an Insurance Professional," Joe Justice Organization, https://www.joejustice.org/tina-white-and-the-importance-of-consulting-an-insurance-professional/.

"Your Source Today," Page 2 of 35, https://yoursourcetoday.com/page/2.

"Community Learning: Utilizing Event Spaces for Group Homeschooling Sessions," Stephanie's Creative Space, 2024, https://stephaniescreativespace.com/community-learning-utilizing-event-spaces-for-group-homeschooling-sessions/.

"The Risks and Rewards of EOM," PatientPoint, May 12, 2023, https://www.patientpoint.com/blog/risks-rewards-eom.

"Maad Labs," https://www.maadlabs.io/strategic-design-kit/problem-tree-analysis.

"Boosting Your E-commerce with WooCommerce CRM Plugin for WordPress," CRM Business Tools, https://crm.teknobgt.com/boosting-your-e-commerce-with-woocommerce-crm-plugin-for-wordpress.

"Nation AI: Unlock the Power of AI with Generative Technology," Nation AI, https://nation.ai/unlock-the-power-of-ai-with-generative-ia-technology/.

"Enhancing Ecommerce Discovery: The Power of Visual Search," September 19, 2023, https://www.visenze.com/blog/2023/09/19/enhancing-ecommerce-discovery-the-power-of-visual-search/.

"Sustainable Development Goals Archives," greenambassadors.org.uk, February 3, 2024, https://greenambassadors.org.uk/tag/sustainable-development-goals/.

"United Arab Emirates: Global Robotic MedTech Forum Concludes Its 1st Edition in Dubai, MENA Report, 2023.

Singh, "Cabinet Health Shark Tank: Transforming Healthcare with Innovative Solutions," July 12, 2023, https://guruvanee.com/cabinet-health-shark-tank/.

"RunBot: Simplifying Location Details in Logistics," RunBuggy, https://runbuggy.com/runbot-simplifying-location-details-in-logistics/.

Macdonald, Kara, "Inman Connect 2023: The Future of Real Estate Wrap Up," Close with Potomac, February 4, 2023, https://www.closewithpotomac.com/inman-connect-new-york-2023-wrap-up/.

"Vitals Capture Archives," Caregility, https://caregility.com/blog/tag/vitals-capture/.

CHAPTER 10

AI WILL CHANGE EVERYTHING, EXCEPT WHAT MATTERS MOST

W e stand on the cusp of a new era in healthcare. AI's transformative potential is undeniable. Integrating AI emerges as a pivotal force reshaping paradigms and practices in the ever-evolving healthcare landscape. The purpose I seek at the heart of this evolving partnership with AI is a truly personalized patient-centered approach to health and healthcare.

As healthcare systems have grown ever larger and more complex, pursuing personalized, holistic care has faced daunting challenges, primarily because of information asymmetry—a situation where one healthcare system or provider network has more or better information than another—and time constraints limiting patient-provider interactions. With AI, this convergence of vast data processing capabilities and ubiquitous technology presents an unprecedented opportunity. Truly personalized healthcare transitions from an impossible aspiration to an attainable reality.

AI's ability to analyze vast datasets, glean insights, conduct genomic analyses, and forecast outcomes can usher in an era of data-driven individualized care. We've mentioned how wearable devices that track daily activities and vital signs can be conduits of real-time, personalized health data, data that informs the provider's treatment plan and provides instant feedback that empowers people to take an active role in managing their own health.

AI enables a level of personalization that was once unimaginable. And better yet we can expect better patient outcomes. This paradigm shift will transcend traditional healthcare settings by effortlessly integrating health management into daily routines. Beyond patient care, AI is catalyzing groundbreaking advancements in biotechnology and drug discovery. AI-enabled genomic analysis is unraveling complex genetic interactions.

AI is transforming every stage of the drug discovery pipeline, from screening potential drug candidates to simulating clinical trial outcomes. AI's prowess in screening potential medication ingredients is already yielding novel treatments and democratizing access to innovation across research domains. Moreover, AI's ability to analyze genomic data unlocks new insights into the underlying disease mechanisms, paving the way for precision medicine and personalized therapies.

Tomorrow's AI Will Dwarf the Best AI of Today

AI can potentially revolutionize every aspect of healthcare delivery, from diagnosis to treatment and beyond. And today's AI represents a mere glimpse of tomorrow's transformative potential. As algorithms become increasingly sophisticated and computing power continues to expand exponentially, the capabilities of AI in healthcare will reach new heights. Tomorrow's AI will analyze data to interpret complex biological phenomena, predict disease trajectories, and tailor interventions with unparalleled precision. The implications of this technological revolution for healthcare are profound, promising to usher in an era of smarter, more efficient, and more effective medical care.

As this evolution unfolds, *The Art of Human Care* becomes ever more important. AI can allow providers to step back from their laptops and truly engage in a conversation. AI can free up hours in a physician's day so they have more time to spend with patients, and office staff can accommodate more people with acute needs. The best marriage of AI and healthcare will nurture relationships, with algorithms turning all those numbers back into names.

One More Look at VP4: Three Pillars Plus

Over my years of service with the Navy, I've had the pleasure of working with Dr. Andrew Plummer. Throughout his career Drew has served as a medical officer and epidemiologist for the US Army and as a captain commissioned officer in the US Public Health Service. For the past decade, he has served as a senior medical advisor and held leadership roles in population health and clinical analytics for the DHA, including a focus on the potential of generative AI in healthcare as the inaugural chair of the DHA Artificial Intelligence Workgroup. An area of interest for years has been how we leverage technology such as AI for situational awareness and decision support for the warfighter and medical professionals on the front lines, particularly in operational medicine and humanitarian assistance contexts. Drew's expertise spans from clinical practice to public health policy, always with an eye toward innovative applications of technology to improve health outcomes particularly in resource scarce environments.

Drew and I often engage in deep discussions about AI and healthcare. We have a penchant for lengthy conversations, using each other as sounding boards for our latest musings on AI and healthcare. The following insights Drew shared with me recently help illustrate how, with AI as our VP, we can truly advance *The Art of Human Care*'s three pillars—purpose, personalization, and partnerships—with the result being increased productivity, i.e., better health outcomes for patients, increased patient throughput in health systems, and higher career satisfaction among providers to deliver smarter healthcare with AI. Here's what Dr. Plummer had to say:

AI and Achieving Our Purpose

We are embarking on the unrealized golden age of biotechnology. For many, many years, we've been talking about the potential of biotech to revolutionize everything from cancer therapy to drug discovery. We're beginning to see some indications of that starting with things like CRISPR,[30] a technology that research scientists use to selectively modify the DNA of living organisms. We're literally editing genes—talk about personal.

AI helps us understand the genome more effectively because we're not only looking at the genes themselves but the gene products, the things that cause them to be activated. We're analyzing that data with AI to understand what's happening at the cellular level with a specific set of genes, how they interact with other genes. It's a lot of data. But it's data that lends itself to fusion and integration as we try to understand what the ultimate outcomes are, the genomics, proteomics—that whole world as opposed to just the gene, the proteins themselves and how they behave in different environments. The folks looking into that are going to utilize AI. AI really provides the rocket fuel to almost any discipline that you can think of.

As far as drug discovery, in December 2023, MIT researchers discovered a new class of antibiotics. With AI, they were able to screen upwards of forty thousand compounds that included most of the known antibiotics as well as a diverse array of molecules, testing each compound for its ability to inhibit the growth of MRSA with methicillin-resistant Staphylococcus aureus, a drug-resistant bacterium that causes more than ten thousand deaths in the United States every year.[31]

There were also 12 million other compounds from a special database, and they were able to screen those. They ended up with about 3,500 antibiotic compounds that had a low toxicity. Then they took a deeper dive and literally came up with a new class of antibiotics to potentially combat MRSA. They wouldn't have been able to do this without AI.

That's just one example of what we're going to see over the next ten years.

What's especially interesting to me is that this won't be confined to the largest pharmaceutical companies. There's some democratization to this process. If you have access to the database and you're a researcher with an idea, this is absolutely powerful.

Many times, you have folks who are working on something novel, but they're not funded enough. Now they have the tools to test their hypothesis.

Even looking at the materials that we use for medical instrumentation, for medical devices, for organs—could AI help us with developing synthetic organs for transplant? That would be a massive win down the road. Fast-forward to a time when the only potential shortage in an organ transplant is having a team to do the procedure as opposed to the actual organ itself.

AI can even simulate clinical trial outcomes or optimize who a trial is based on. AI can be very balanced and ethical in ensuring diversity, equity, and inclusion so trial results will have representation of underserved communities.

AI Making It Personal

In medicine, we aim to offer a patient-centered approach to health and healthcare. This is aspirational. From a historical perspective and from a technical perspective, it's what we try to do. It's obviously a laudable goal. It's challenging to do at scale because of everything from asymmetry to the amount of information available for an individual patient. There is an unspoken expectation that the provider is aware of all the factors that might impact not only that specific episode of care but also care going forward—that engagement will inform what's likely to happen in the future. This is this idea of a personalized, patient-centered, holistic approach that includes everything from the health status of the patient from a behavioral health and physical perspective to their environmental and social determinants of health.

There are many things that happen outside of a patient's visit with their provider. The time a patient is in front of them and when they're speaking to the patient is the time they have available to influence a patient, and it's an extremely small percentage of time.

I think about where we are today. We have that combination of the ability to process massive amounts of data and the proximity of technology available to the patient, i.e., a mobile phone in their hand or mobile, wearable devices that are collecting information, and our ability to store, process, and analyze more and more information.

This puts us in a special place. We have the opportunity to move from an aspiration to a realization of personalized, patient-centered, holistic care.

AI as a Partner

If you asked me five years ago, I would have said we're missing a key ingredient to tie all this together. It's not that we weren't using AI and machine learning specifically. But now, with AI, we have algorithms that can forecast and provide us with descriptive epidemiology. They can tell us, "By the way, you got this many steps" and "Hey, you're sleeping better. You are in bed earlier, you're sleeping longer, and it looks like you don't wake up quite as much." Maybe that meant that you lost some weight, and your sleep apnea has improved. You're literally going to draw conclusions based on that data analysis.

Let's take a look at some more variables—the number of steps you walked every day, the calories you took in, the number of times you got up from your seat, and how many times your watch reminded you to take a deep breath.

A good study has many individuals. Researchers try to get the right sample size to be able to say whether statistically there was a difference. Personally, am I interested in what happens to the cohort? No, I'm more concerned about how my behavior has changed my sleep. In order to do that at a population level, you're talking about a big study whereas I can learn a lot about myself because of the many, many data points that are collected by my devices over long periods of time.

This is where AI is special. The big idea here is that we're going to be able to review significant amounts of data. We're going to be able to analyze that data. And we're going to be able to draw inferences from that data even if it's individual, not part of some specific study. It's on one individual. We're able to read over their longitudinal data and draw some conclusions.

With AI, when you establish the baselines, you can set some goals that you'd like to meet from a health perspective. Maybe you are working with a medical provider, a nutritionist, a physical therapist, a psychologist or psychiatrist, or a health coach. Now whatever it was that they were encouraging you to do, you have the opportunity to track the instructions and to track the outcomes.

For example, if I'm supposed to be on a low-sodium diet, I'm hypertensive, or I'm in the gray zone, we go to an app, record the sorts of foods that I'm eating, and track that as one mechanism to reduce sodium. Take it another step, we ask the app about a diet or lifestyle change that will reduce sodium as a routine part of my daily nutrition, and it gives me a week's worth of recipes, making it easy to stick to that goal.

There's an application that can shop for those foods for you via Instacart, as an example, and even have it delivered. You've gone from this idea, this personalized recommendation from a professional, to an eating plan that is congruent with that goal, and you don't have to leave your desk because your groceries will arrive. When you think of the friction that's been removed, not only the physical friction but the cognitive friction, that's special. That's when we're getting into this idea of personalized health.

If I'm a patient with a Fitbit, a scale that measures my weight, or a blood pressure cuff that transmits information, if I can get that information in my personal health records seamlessly and safely, then the systems are going to embrace that information, and they're going to utilize it in a constructive way. On the other side, providers in the care team are able to take that information and generate this personalized approach.

If there's a single standard that would allow me to share my information when I'm not even at my local hospital, when I'm on vacation, AI could facilitate an analysis and summary of that data wherever I show up with it. I have my information on my watch, for example.

Wearable technologies will continue to evolve. For example, they can track things like the heart rate, the characteristics of an individual's heart rate at rest or when they're walking or exercising. That's one example. But to be able to do that across a plethora of variables, like blood sugar, for example, that's a hot one, right? As they continually monitor your glucose, you begin to appreciate how the time of day, the types of foods, even your mood can kick off a cascade of metabolic implications.

As we become more sophisticated at extracting information that really describes me as an individual, it becomes super powerful, and it begins to correlate outcomes with this data. When we start to scale that up to groups of individuals, then communities, and then populations, we begin to potentially see trends and signals that may be important for population health and for disease prevention.

We'll likely get to the point where we are aware of levels of medications in our blood and can learn the best time of day to take a medication based on an individual and who they are.

A device that collects information about weather and air quality has implications for a child who has asthma. The school nurse and teachers can decide to have that child to sit out of some activities. This all comes back to this personalized approach, not a one-size-fits-all.

So the healthcare system has collected my genome, my biomarkers, my vital signs, my habits. Now what about privacy, ethics, security, and safety? That is going to be extremely important because they know a lot about me. But if used appropriately, this is a great thing because we can co-create positive health outcomes—myself, my provider, and the system. This is the aha moment, the eureka moment.

A patient moves from the contemplative phase all the way to the action phase when they recognize that there's something in it for them. The ability to have a dialogue, to experience the outcomes, awareness of the outcomes—I think this knowledge is going to change things in the next ten years. And I think the engagement between the patient and their healthcare provider is going to be almost continuous but not in an overbearing way. There will certainly be a lot more action in the white space between office visits than there is today.

We will have the ability to use the healthcare system to promote health as opposed to treating poor health. By far, this is the most important capability—to promote health. Especially if these routines and expectations are ingrained at a young age. When my son wears a Fitbit, and he thinks it's just what people do, it's a routine thing.

Within the next decade, the thing that stands out to me most with regard to AI's potential is the ability of the patient to be a more active contributor to their own health outcomes. If we really merge and fuse the data and concurrently encourage the patient to do the things that will help them meet health goals, the literature suggests this will result in ideal outcomes at both individual and population levels. They're going to have access to more information than they've ever had before. They're going to have access to more individual personal information than ever before. And they're going to be able to marry all of that to optimize their own health outcomes. That is where I see us going within the next ten years.

It's not only access to information but actionable knowledge that is self-directed.

It's about that dialogue in the white space. I really haven't heard anybody talking about it this way, but that's how I think about it. It's a continuous engagement that is self-directed most of the time because patients have opted in in a nonintrusive way. It potentially becomes the standard. It includes everything from the obvious like making an appointment to see a provider with a phone, or doing something without having to call a provider like picking up a prescription, or having it delivered before it runs out. Patients don't miss a beat. And they're compliant with their medication. And perhaps it's even adjusted because their blood pressure is now under control. Their provider knows this because they've been sharing blood pressure readings and perhaps with a virtual call. It's data driven and cocreated with the provider.

A significant number of folks aren't going to have to go into the office for care. Time is valuable as a human being, as a patient, and as a provider.

AI, Productivity, and Survival

Something the military has been bullish on for years is seeing the warfighter as an athlete—if you're special forces, an elite athlete. Ideally, we're optimizing their health and well-being so that they are ready to fight tonight, ready to deploy anytime, anywhere. There is this idea of a medically ready force to support the warfighter on the ground, often because of limitations that we can all appreciate..

Of course, this always brings up concerns around privacy and security, particularly in the military where there are concerns about operational security risks associated with the free flow of information. Many industries, like the banking industry, for example, have successfully navigated those waters. If we couldn't trust the banking system and our banking transactions, we'd be stuck. We know that it's possible to securely enter personalized financial information, like credit card numbers or bank account routing numbers in a public place and be successful and not get hacked as long as you've got a VPN or something similar.

In the military, point-of-injury care is a very, very serious concern. A scenario where a combination of factors like temperature, oxygen saturation, heart rate, other variables suggests that maybe it's time to end a drill or an exercise because we may see some heat injuries or other negative outcomes associated with training in an austere environment.

AI can also reduce the administrative burden for the provider, bringing the joy back to medicine, reducing the cognitive burden on the provider, while at the same time maintaining his or her autonomy in the process.

What Matters Most

AI assumes a dual role in military healthcare, optimizing warfighter readiness and ensuring operational security. By leveraging AI-driven health monitoring, military units prioritize soldier well-being, mitigate risks, and enhance operational effectiveness. However, privacy concerns underscore the imperative of robust security safeguards in data management.

The transformative impact will reverberate globally as AI permeates every facet of military and civilian healthcare. From personalized medicine to biotechnological breakthroughs, AI propels healthcare into an unparalleled era of innovation and collaboration. Embracing AI's potential means we must navigate ethical, privacy, and security considerations to build a future where healthcare is not reactive but proactive. A future that empowers individuals with data sovereignty to reclaim agency over their health and well-being.

I retired from military service in the summer of 2023. On a very warm day in July of that year, I stood before the assembled guests of my retirement party to deliver my speech, marking the culmination of twenty-five years of dedicated naval service. Despite initial resistance to the idea of a retirement ceremony, wise counsel from a great friend, Dr. James Cowan, led me to embrace the celebration of my service as a tribute not to myself but rather to my wife, son, daughter, family, and friends who supported me over every day of my service.

As I began my address, an unexpected power outage plunged the venue into darkness, leaving the room lit only by a setting sun. The sweltering summer heat added to the discomfort. Undeterred, my voice rang out without a microphone. I began by reciting the "Preamble to the US Constitution," a timeless reminder of the principles that had guided my career and life.

"We, the people of the United States, in order to form a more perfect Union, establish justice, ensure domestic tranquility, provide for the common defense, promote the general welfare, and secure the blessings of Liberty to ourselves and our posterity, do ordain and establish this Constitution for the United States of America."

I went on to share anecdotes and reflections, recounting my journey from the moment I raised my hand to support and defend the Constitution and accepted a commission in the United States Navy. While reflecting on pivotal moments in my career without the ability to display the planned photo slide show and videos, I shared humorous anecdotes, such as that unexpected assignment to the aircraft carrier USS *Carl Vinson* (CVN-70) as a new "green" surgeon on my first operational deployment. Despite my challenges, I remained steadfast in embodying the Navy's principles of honor, courage, and commitment throughout my twenty-two months on the ship and nineteen months at sea.

Appropriately, at the climax of my speech, I turned my attention to my family and highlighted their profound impact on my life and career. From my son's strong and steadfast ambition to attend Georgetown Preparatory School to my daughter's quiet courage and creative artistic flair through her years at Stone Ridge School of the Sacred Heart, I spoke of their love and resilience as an inspiration that defined our relationships.

I acknowledged my wife's unwavering support and shared how we renewed our twenty-year vows just days before the retirement ceremony, reaffirming our commitment to each other amid the inevitable challenges we faced as a couple.

As I reflected on the concept of service, I shared a poignant encounter with a young man who thanked me for my service. This highlighted the profound impact and role of the US military in preserving the ideals enshrined in the Constitution. Drawing parallels between the preamble and that young man's experiences, I again emphasized to all those in attendance the importance of serving to uphold the principles of justice, domestic tranquility, and the common defense.

Despite the power outage and the discomfort it brought, the ordeal as it unfolded revealed what truly matters most—deep human connection. Though spoken in the absence of amplification, electricity, and light, I was informed that my words resonated deeply with the audience, creating an atmosphere of love, fellowship, and friendship that transcended the uncomfortable physical surroundings. As my guests listened intently in the darkness, a sense of camaraderie filled the room, moving everyone in attendance and testifying to the shared humanity that binds us together.

AI's implications for healthcare are far reaching, touching every aspect of the healthcare ecosystem. From remote patient monitoring to telemedicine platforms, AI can facilitate delivering high-quality healthcare services to underserved populations and remote regions.

As AI continues to reshape the healthcare landscape, our humanity must inform the ethical, societal, and regulatory challenges that arise. From ensuring patient privacy and data security to addressing algorithmic bias, ensuring algorithmic equity, and transparency issues, the moral implications of AI in healthcare are complex and multifaceted. Moreover, we must take brave steps to ensure regulatory frameworks evolve to keep pace with the rapid advancements in AI technology. AI-driven healthcare solutions must be safe, effective, and equitable.

So yeah, AI will change and impact everything except the things that matter most. Indeed, the things that matter most and serve to connect us as humans—love, friendship, fellowship, and care—will endure even in the darkness and uncertainty of our AI future.

NOTES

Lekkala, L. R., "How AI Analytical Models Can Use FHIR (Fast Healthcare Interoperability Resources) Data," *Voice of the Publisher* 9, no. 4 (December 2023), https://doi.org/10.4236/vp.2023.94016.

"10 Ways Wearable Technology Transforms the Healthcare," Techovedas, November 14, 2023, https://techovedas. com/10-ways-wearable-technology-transforms-the-healthcare/.

"Awais Awe," Author at Longevity LIVE, https://longevitylive.com/author/awais-awe/.

"Ethics of AI in Law: Addressing Bias, Privacy, Transparency," July 8, 2024, https://www.indikaai.com/blog/the-ethics-of-ai-in-the-legal-industry-2.

"Case Discussion on Precision Care after Cardiac Arrest," Pooja Wadwa, Assimilate by Medvarsity, https://assimilate.one/case-discussion/case-discussion-on-precision-care-after-cardiac-arrest/.

Turner, M., Aspin, G., Didymus, F., Mack, R., Olusoga, P., Wood, A., and Bennett, R., "One Case, Four Approaches: The Application of Psychotherapeutic Approaches in Sport Psychology," *The Sport Psychologist* 34, no. 1 (March 2020), https://doi.org/10.1123/tsp.2019-0079.

"Pharmabackoffice," Immunechem, https://immunechem.com/author/pharmabackoffice/.

"AI-Powered Medical Devices Revolutionize Healthcare Diagnosis and Treatment," https://ushandyman.net/ai-powered-medical-devices-revolutionize-healthcare-diagnosis-and-treatment/.

"Vitals Capture Archives," Caregility, https://caregility.com/blog/tag/vitals-capture/.

"Human-Centered Design in Healthcare IT," Code Power, January 10, 2024, https://www.codepwr.com/human-centered-design-in-healthcare/.

Katri, Nishan, "Artificial Intelligence in Healthcare: Improving Patient Care," November 29, 2023, https://nishankhatri.xyz/artificial-intelligence-in-healthcare-improving-patient-care/.

"5 Ways GPT-4 Transforms Business, Insights, and Applications," Fluid22, 2024, https://fluid22.com/insights/unlocking-business-potential-with-gpt-4-a-fluid22-perspective.

"The Future of Renewable Energy in Comoros: Exploring Wind Power Potential | REVE News of the Wind Sector in Spain and in the World," July 1, 2023, https://www.evwind.es/2023/07/01/the-future-of-renewable-energy-in-comoros-exploring-wind-power-potential/92561.

Safa, "Artificial Intelligence: A New Era of Innovation," February 12, 2015, https://club-admiral-777.net/unleashing-the-potential-of-artificial-intelligence-a-new-era-of-innovation/.

"What Is the Most Important Goal of the Constitution?" Tracks-movie.com, https://tracks-movie.com/what-is-the-most-important-goal-of-the-constitution/.

ACKNOWLEDGMENTS

First, this book would not exist without the service, care, sacrifice, and compassion of all who have cared for another human. I am incredibly thankful for those who work every day in our places of healing, especially in the military, to do the hard work of restoring health and wellness and for the innovators who bring us new technology to do our work better. These individuals deserve all the honor.

I am indebted to the many patients I met and cared for over the years, for they provided inspiration and wisdom. Robert Pearl's *ChatGPT, MD: How AI-Empowered Patients & Doctors Can Take Back Control of American Medicine* provided invaluable context to characterize AI and healthcare for the zeitgeist. Special thanks to my research advisors and mentors at the National War College, John W. Yaeger, Kelly Ward, and John Via. Additionally, thanks to Ritu Agarwal, Amy Brown, James Cimino, Christopher Dewing, Kevin Dorrance, Eric Elster, Heather Flannery, Andy Gettinger, Matt Goldman, Christyl Johnson, Amol Joshi, Caesar Junker, Ryan Kappadel, Arthur Kellerman, Rebecca Lee, Danyelle Long, Michael Malanoski, Karen Matthews, Scott McKeithen, Nand Mulchandani, Niels Olson, Michelle Padgett, Andrew Plummer, Charles Rice, Adam

Robinson, David Sontag, Pete Walker, and Jonathan Woodson for their invaluable contributions and for sharing their thoughts and perspectives on AI and medicine.

My teachers, mentors, and coaches have directly and indirectly influenced this work and taught me the healing art of medicine. The conceptual, editorial, and creative work of Bettina Experton, Thomas Moran, Jeremy Pamplin, Joe Pardavilla, Stoney Trent, Karen McDiarmid, Estelle Slootmaker, Severence MacLaughlin, Jack Canfield, Colin Powell, Michael Groen, Lieutenant General (USMC, Retired), John 'Jack' Shanahan, Lieutenant General (USAF, Retired), Uhura Chartered Corporation, and the Forbes Books team was priceless.

Finally, the most thanks must go to my family, especially my wife Lisa, son Edmund, and daughter Ella, who tolerate and support both a surgeon's and an author's schedule. Thank you all for always listening at the kitchen table to endless recitals, for enduring many drafts and revisions, and for your patience, love, and support with tea, a special treat, and warm embrace through many days and long nights. You are all a blessing I am fortunate to have, and I thank God for you every day.

Hassan A. Tetteh, MD
Washington, DC

OTHER BOOKS BY

DR. HASSAN A. TETTEH

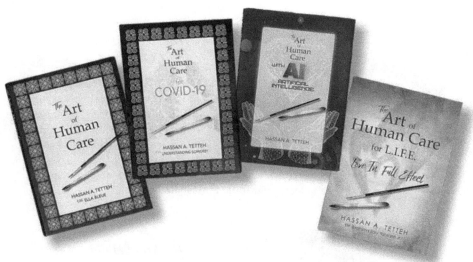

The Art of Human Care® Series

The Art of Human Care theory embodies Purpose, Personalization, and Partnerships. Inspired by his near-death experience and informed over decades of clinical practice as a heart and lung transplant surgeon, Dr. Tetteh combines many of his personal stories with the healing power of art. His down-to-earth humanitarianism and unique perspective on what it means to heal serves to inspire individuals to change the world positively.

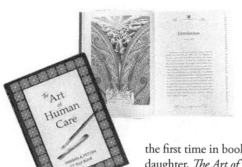

The Art of Human Care

In 2014, Dr. Hassan A. Tetteh delivered a deeply inspiring speech to first-year medical students during their White Coat Ceremony at his medical school alma mater. Now, published for the first time in book form with illustrations from his daughter, *The Art of Human Care* presents Tetteh's words of wisdom and answers the question: How can we change the world through healing?

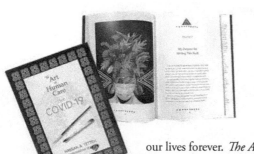

The Art of Human Care for COVID-19

The Art of Human Care for COVID-19 can positively change your life. The global COVID-19 pandemic claimed countless lives, impacted the world, and changed our lives forever. *The Art of Human Care for COVID-19* serves to answer this question: How can we positively change our world through healing?

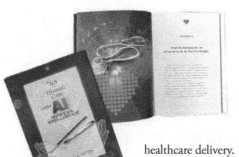

The Art of Human Care with Artificial Intelligence

The Art of Human Care with Artificial Intelligence prepares you for the future. The AI revolution is here. AI is fundamentally changing the landscape of healthcare delivery. *The Art of Human Care with AI* serves to answer the question: How can we leverage AI to change our world through healing?

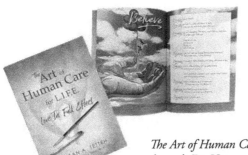

The Art of Human Care for L.I.F.E.—Love in Full Effect

The Art of Human Care for L.I.F.E. defines Human Care with art and love. The acronym L.I.F.E. stands for Love In Full Effect. This special edition in *The Art of Human Care* book series expresses this theme through Dr. Hassan A. Tetteh's own stories of healing and inspiration that are adeptly infused with the healing power of art and his own poetry. Overall, the book calls on us to look to love as we each work to positively make changes in the world.

Other books by Dr. Hassan A. Tetteh

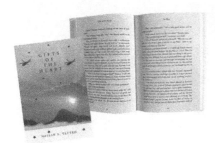

Gifts of the Heart

Hassan Tetteh's powerful novel is an inspiration and a gift. Dr. Kareem Afram, a young military physician and heart surgeon, comes of age in the desert of Afghanistan. He overcomes trials, challenges, destruction, illness, and death to accomplish the impossible and provide a blueprint for living one's life to the fullest.

The story of the doctor lures you in with riveting scenes of life-and-death hospital emergencies and combat surgery, but it is in learning about the doctor's life that causes you to stay and get comfortable. You will encounter reflections of your own character, flaws, strengths, and vulnerability. As you stay for the journey and share in the doctor's life, you learn of triumph over struggle and see reflections of your strength, your power, your will, and your own conviction to ask yourself life's most urgent question. The message within is universal, a gift of the heart, an education in freedom, and touches your soul to make an undeniable impression that stays long after the last page is turned.

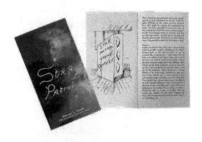

Star Patrol

An invitation to be a TEDx speaker in 2019 provided Dr. Tetteh with the opportunity to revisit his *Star Patrol* 'book,' written at age twelve for a Young Authors' Festival in New York City. *Star Patrol* is republished in its original format with a foreword written by Dr. Tetteh's son, Edmund E. Tetteh. The twelve-year-old author from Brooklyn dreams about the future and describes a heroic crime fighter. Like *Star Patrol*'s hero, Dr. Tetteh turned a passion into a purpose, and works every day to make the impossible possible and save the world one patient at a time.

ENDNOTES

1   "Suicide Data and Statistics," CDC, accessed July 2, 2024, https://www.cdc.gov/suicide/facts/data.html.

2   Farzana Akkas, "Youth Suicide Risk Increased over Past Decade," Pew, March 3, 2023, https://www.pewtrusts.org/en/research-and-analysis/articles/2023/03/03/youth-suicide-risk-increased-over-past-decade.

3   David Jin et al., "Independent Assessment of a Deep Learning System for Lymph Node Metastasis Detection on the Augmented Reality Microscope," *Journal of Pathology Informatics* 13 (2022), https://www.sciencedirect.com/journal/journal-of-pathology-informatics.

4   "Sailor of the Year 20231 Changed How the Navy Dealt with COVID-19," Navy Times, August 25, 2021, https://www.navytimes.com/military-honor/smoy/2021/08/25/this-sailor-ran-covid-testing-on-guam-for-the-uss-teddy-roosevelt-and-changed-how-the-navy-dealt-with-the-virus/.

5   "Anatomic Pathology Digital Whole Slide Scanning Services," University of Iowa, accessed July 2, 2024, https://medicine.uiowa.edu/pathology/node/4721; "Digital and Computational Pathology," Ohio State University, accessed July 2, 2024, https://cancer.osu.edu/for-patients-and-caregivers/learn-about-cancers-and-treatments/clinical-services-at-the-james/digital-pathology/services.

6   "Invisible Wounds Initiative," Air Force Wounded Warrior Program, accessed July 2, 2024, https://www.woundedwarrior.af.mil/airmen-veterans/invisible-wounds-initiative/.

7   "MHS Genesis: The Electronic Health Record," Military Health System, accessed July 2, 2024, https://www.health.mil/Military-Health-Topics/Technology/MHS-GENESIS.

8   Patricia Kime, "VA Halts Future Launches of Its Oracle Cerner Health Record System," Military.com, April 21, 2023, https://www.military.com/daily-news/2023/04/21/troubled-va-medical-records-system-wont-be-added-new-hospitals-anytime-soon-va-halts-rollout.html.

9   "International Classification of Diseases," CDC, accessed July 2, 2024, https://www.cdc.gov/nchs/icd/icd10cm_pcs_background.htm#:~:text=Code%20set%20differences,categories%20instead%20of%20numeric%20ones.

10   "Suicide Data and Statistics," CDC, accessed July 2, 2024, https://www.cdc.gov/suicide/facts/data.html

11   "Army Study to Assess Risk and Resilience in Servicemembers," National Institute of Mental Health, https://www.nimh.nih.gov/research/research-funded-by-nimh/research-initiatives/army-study-to-assess-risk-and-resilience-in-servicemembers-army-starrs.

12   "Suicide Risk and Risk of Death among Recent Veterans," US Department of Veterans Affairs, accessed July 2, 2024, https://www.publichealth.va.gov/epidemiology/studies/suicide-risk-death-risk-recent-veterans.asp.

13   Allan Ripp, "How AI Will Make Your Doctor Smarter," *Wall Street Journal*, November 5, 2021, https://www.wsj.com/articles/how-artificial-intelligence-will-make-your-doctor-smarter-tetteh-medicine-military-covid-ai-11636123757.

14 "National Veteran Suicide Prevention Annual Report 2022," Office of Mental Health and Suicide Prevention, September 2022, https://www.mentalhealth.va.gov/docs/data-sheets/2022/2022-National-Veteran-Suicide-Prevention-Annual-Report-FINAL-508.pdf.

15 "Suicide Data and Statistics," CDC, accessed July 2, 2024, https://www.cdc.gov/suicide/facts/data.html.

16 "Death among Children and Adolescents," Medicine Plus, accessed July 2, 2024, https://medlineplus.gov/ency/article/001915.htm#:~:text=Accidents%20(unintentional%20injuries)%20are%2C,death%20among%20children%20and%20teens.

17 Mario Aquilar, "A 988 Operator, Faced with a Flood of Calls, Turns to AI to Boost Counselor Skills," STAT, June 22, 2023, https://www.statnews.com/2023/06/22/988-suicide-hotline-lyssn-protocall-artificial-intelligence/.

18 Paul Boyce, "Battlefield Medicine and the Urgency to Save Soldiers," US Army, April 26, 2011, https://www.army.mil/article/55508/battlefield_medicine_and_the_urgency_to_save_soldiers.

19 LTCOL Charles H. C. Pilgrim et al., "Treatment at Point of Injury—Forward Movement of Surgical Assets to Address Non-Compressible Truncal Haemorrhage," *Journal of Military and Veterans' Health* 30, no. 1, https://jmvh.org/article/treatment-at-point-of-injury-forward-movement-of-surgical-assets-to-address-non-compressible-truncal-haemorrhage/.

20 Olivia F. Hunter et al., "Science Fiction or Clinical Reality: A Review of the Applications of Artificial Intelligence Along the Continuum of Trauma," *World Journal of Emergency Surgery*, 2023, carehttps://www.ncbi.nlm.nih.gov/pmc/articles/PMC9987401/#:~:text=Starting%20at%20the%20point%20of,inform%20transfer%20location%20and%20urgency.

21 Alexander, George A., "The History—and Future—of Combat Care," June 26, 2018, https://www.ausa.org/articles/history%E2%80%94and-future%E2%80%94-combat-care.

22 Gunst, Mark, et al., "Changing epidemiology of trauma deaths leads to bimodal distribution," *Proceedings (Baylor University Medical Center)* 23, no. 4 (October 2010): 349–354. doi: 10.1080/08998280.2010.11928649.

23 Moore, Charles et al., "A Review of 75th Ranger Regiment Battle-Injured Fatalities Incurred During Combat Operations From 2001 to 2021," *Military Medicine* 189, no. 7-8 (July/August 2024): 1728–1737, doi: https://doi.org/10.1093/milmed/usad331.

24 Rashid, Adib, et al., "Artificial Intelligence in the Military: An Overview of the Capabilities, Applications, and Challenges," International Journal of Intelligent Systems (November 2023), doi: https://doi.org/10.1155/2023/8676366.

25 Matthew Bradley, et al., "Combat casualty care and lessons learned from the past 100 years of war," *Current Problems in Surgery* 54, no. 6, 315-351, https://doi.org/10.1067/j.cpsurg.2017.02.004.

26 Matt McGough et al., "Child and Teen Firearm Mortality in the US and Peer Countries," KFF, July 18, 2023, https://www.kff.org/mental-health/issue-brief/child-and-teen-firearm-mortality-in-the-u-s-and-peer-countries/.

27 Stephen Luchter, Andrew Smith, and Jing Wang, "Fatal Injuries in Light Vehicle Crashes—Time to Death and Cause of Death," *Annual Proceedings of the Association for the Advancement of Automotive Medicine*, 1998, https://www.ncbi.nlm.nih.gov/pmc/articles/PMC3400203/#:~:text=Approximately%2030%20percent%20of%20the,hemorrhage%20or%20severe%20blood%20loss.

28   "Quick Safety 51: Proactive Prevention of Maternal Death
     from Maternal Hemorrhage," Joint Commission, https://www.
     jointcommission.org/resources/news-and-multimedia/newsletters/
     newsletters/quick-safety/quick-safety-issue-51-proactive-
     prevention-of-maternal-death-from-maternal-hemorrhage/
     quick-safety-51-proactive-prevention-of-maternal-death-from-
     maternal-hemorrhage/#:~:text=5%20Approximately%20
     3%2D5%25%20of,will%20experience%20a%20postpartum%20
     hemorrhage.&text=These%20preventable%20events%20are%20
     the,11.2%25%20of%20U.S.%20maternal%20deaths.

29   Beauchamp, T. L., & Childress, J. F. (1979). Principles of
     Biomedical Ethics. Oxford: Oxford University Press

30   "CRISPR," National Human Genome Research Institute,
     last updated July 2, 2024, https://www.genome.gov/genetics-
     glossary/CRISPR#:~:text=CRISPR%20(short%20for%20
     %E2%80%9Cclustered%20regularly,editing%20systems%20
     found%20in%20bacteria.

31   Anne Trafton, "Using AI, MIT Researchers Identify
     a New Class of Antibiotic Candidates," MIT News,
     December 20, 2023, https://news.mit.edu/2023/
     using-ai-mit-researchers-identify-antibiotic-candidates-1220.